EARLY EDUCATION OF AFRICAN AMERICAN PHARMACISTS 1870–1975

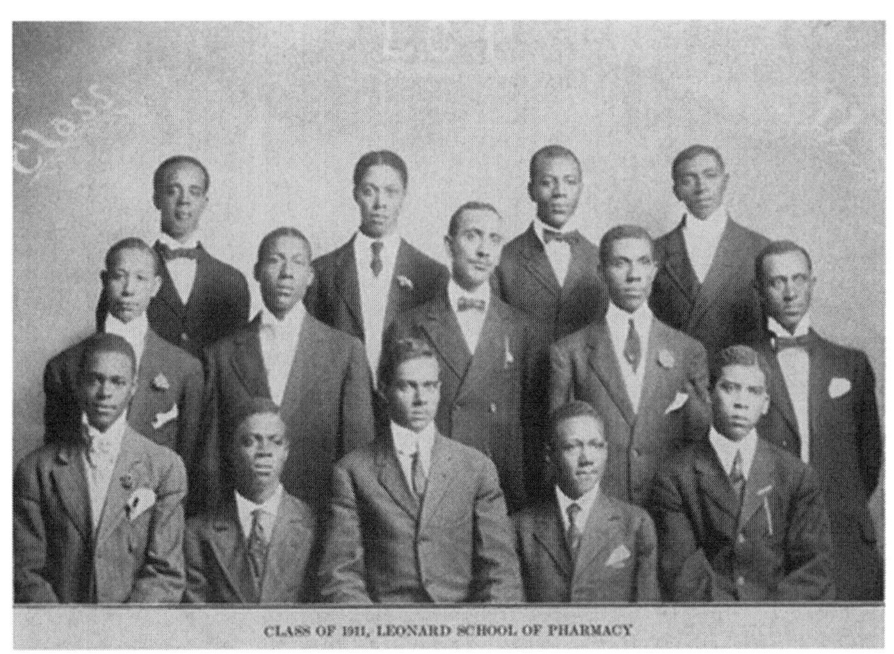

CLASS OF 1911, LEONARD SCHOOL OF PHARMACY

JOHN E. CLARK

EARLY EDUCATION OF AFRICAN AMERICAN PHARMACISTS 1870–1975

BY

JOHN E. CLARK

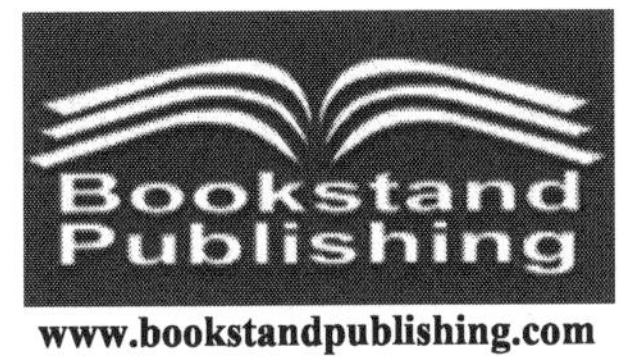

www.bookstandpublishing.com

Published by
Bookstand Publishing
Pasadena, CA 91101
4763_11

ISBN 978-1-63498-913-8

Library of Congress Control Number: 2020909170

Table of Contents

List of Tables

List of Figures

Contributors

Diane S. Allen-Gipson, Ph.D., M.S.
Tenured Associate Professor, Department of Pharmaceutical Sciences, University of South Florida, Taneja College of Pharmacy, Tampa, Florida

Angela M. Hill, Pharm.D., CRPh
Professor & Associate Dean of Clinical Affairs, Taneja College of Pharmacy, University of South Florida, Tampa, Florida

Trudy Kelly, MLS
Reference Librarian
St. Petersburg College, St. Petersburg, Florida

Ira Charles Robinson, Ph.D., R.Ph.
Professor of Pharmacy, Former Dean College of Pharmacy, Florida A&M University, Tallahassee, Florida, Former Dean College of Pharmacy, Howard University, Washington, D.C.

Raisah Salhab, Pharm.D.
Clinical Pharmacist, Red Crescent Clinic of Tampa Bay, BRIDGE Healthcare Clinic, Tampa, Florida

Sarah J. Steinhardt, Pharm.D., J.D., M.S.
Assistant Professor, Department of Pharmacotherapeutics and Clinical Research, University of South Florida, Taneja College of Pharmacy, Tampa, Florida

Deborah E. Williams, M.D., Ph.D., M.S.
Curriculum Phase II Director, Associate Professor of Pathology, Rowan University School of Osteopathic Medicine, Stratford, New Jersey

Foreword

There are no events that happen per chance and with every event there is predestine action to come forth. In celebrating Woman's History month, nothing could have predicted where my inquiry would lead regarding "who were the pioneers for women in pharmacy." More specifically, were there any African American women pioneers in pharmacy. After several calls to colleagues, it led me to the author Dr. John Clark. As a result of our conversation it unearths the presence in history of phenomenal black women in pharmacy whom during the antebellum south continued to make history. As leaders these women during segregation and Jim Crow shaped history and illuminate the challenges they faced. As professionals they were ostracized by the AMA (American Medical Association) because of race and gender. Believing to find solace in the sisterhood, the suffrage movement revealed their overarching platform for women's rights could not be separated from embracing the oxymoron separate and not equal. The preparation of this manuscript has been a work of love in which the author tells the story of his profession and his people. The collection of newspaper articles, photos and data to support understanding the educational and professional evolution of these courageous *Sojourner Truth* heroes testifies to their greatness. Over time the story evolved from the focus on the women to the focus on the educational institutions that made their success possible. Under the veil of history, the author finds the seeds of health disparities. The basket weaving of information leads to the rationale for the paucity of African American physicians and pharmacist buried in the Flexner report. Dr. Abraham Flexner, educator and critic, has the dubious distinction of offering the 1908 appraisal of *The American College: A Criticism*. As a result of his critical document on American education the Carnegie Foundation commissioned Dr. Flexner to survey 155 medical colleges in the U.S. and Canada. The Flexner report served as the accreditation standard that pivoted the closure of countless African American medical schools and Colleges of pharmacy. These educational institutions not only provide the opportunity for African American to gain professional education but provide the human resource to service a community ignored by white physicians and pharmacists. The early African American women pioneers in pharmacy attended many of these schools. Without them…. and the impact they had many of us would not be here with the ability to stand on their shoulders. They made enormous contributions to the pharmacy profession and pharmacy education but they leverage a socio-political impact in changing the tide of racism across the country. They supported political engagement through advocacy and channeled resources from pharmacy businesses to help others within the field and outside the field to create a greater economic base for African Americans.

It is my hope that this book will reveal to the reader an appreciation and respect for our past champions and what we must do in the future to honor their legacy. The more we learn about our history the more our purpose in the future is revealed. The information compiled in this book is reflective of the contribution of so many nationwide. It is with endearing grace that the author thanks all contributors those mentioned and not mentioned. But much more needs to be written for the story is more than a mile wide and an inch deep. This book reflects the beginning … that our journey to the promised land will be as a community and not by individual effort. This is our heritage, this is their gift to us.

Deborah E. Williams, M.D., Ph.D., MS
Curriculum Phase II Director
Associate Professor of Pathology
Rowan University School of Osteopathic Medicine
Stratford, New Jersey

Acknowledgements

There are so many people who have given me inspiration and support at different stages of the writing of this book that I am almost afraid to mention names for fear that I may overlook someone. The person who gave me the initial inspiration to pursue this project was my dear friend Dr. Deborah Williams. I first met Deborah over the telephone when she was Associate Professor of Pathology at the Touro College of Pharmacy in New York. Our conversation culminated in her asking me if I knew who was the first African American female pharmacist in America. Because I was uncertain who that might be, I started searching the literature and the internet, which led me to the early defunct pharmacy schools that I knew very little about. Her critical thoughts and keen sense of medical history have been invaluable in helping guide me through the thought process for this project. I give special thanks and appreciation to Dr. William Kelly and his wife Mrs. Trudy Kelly for their advice, editorial assistance, and inspiration. Dr. Kevin Sneed, Senior Associate Vice-President, USF Health, Professor and Dean, and Dr. Angela Hill, Professor and Associate Dean of Clinical Affairs, University of South Florida, Taneja College of Pharmacy have been my phenomenal and greatest cheerleaders. I would like to acknowledge the assistance of the following individuals for their advice, guidance, editing, and identification, and for the collecting of the historical information used to write this manuscript: Dr. Gregory Bond, Dr. Stephen Greenberg, Dr. Todd Savitt, Dr. Ira Robinson, Miss Kayla Mackanin, and Mrs. Mary K. Marlatt at the University of Louisville library.

Preface

The interest in research, education, science, and medicine has always been at the forefront of the study of history in the U.S. While there has been some attention given to African American physicians, nurses, chemists, and scientists, less focus has been on the history of African American pharmacists and the segregated defunct pharmacy schools where many first received their early education and training. It is uncertain why this attention has been lacking. Perhaps it is because of a lack of awareness, interest, disregard, or deliberate omission of historical information about the early education of African American pharmacists. While gathering information about this intriguing topic, one may get the impression that because the early black pharmacy schools were forced to close, they may not have been seen by the pharmacy community as being worthy of their support, even to service their own community. Because they were seen by many of their professional colleagues, and the public, as illegitimate, perhaps it was felt that historical discussion was not warranted, even though the churches and some religious organizations strongly supported them. Graduates of the schools were perceived as inferior and indifferent by other pharmacists. They were also not trusted and were thought to be incompetent.

Records of most of the defunct pharmacy programs, which could give a better understanding of their curriculums, training, faculty, and students, were treated with little significance and importance because so much of the information has been lost or destroyed. Therefore, making such information about the schools extremely difficult to find. If not for some stories being told and newspaper accounts, it would almost appear as if these schools never existed. Perhaps that was the intent as it became all too common for details about the pharmacy programs, as well as their accomplishments and challenges, to be omitted from stories of American history.

My early interest in this topic was piqued by the publications of Todd L. Savitt, "Four African American Proprietary Medical Colleges: 1888-1923," in the *Journal of the History of Medical Allied Sciences,* 55.3 (2000). Dr. Savitt focused on the early defunct African American medical schools. As he took a close look at the medical school's programs, administration, and their challenges, it became clear and very intriguing that most all the early pharmacy programs were departments of the early black medical schools. Although his work makes mention of the pharmacy departments, it does not provide detailed information about the programs' characteristics, faculty, students, degrees offered, or the curriculum.

The information provided by Chauncey I. Cooper: "Section 12. The Negro in Pharmacy," in *The General Report of the Pharmaceutical Survey 1946-49*, ed. Edward C. Elliott (Washington, DC: American Council on Education, 1947), helped guide the direction taken in this book by providing a very compelling argument and discussion about the purpose and significance of the early African American pharmacy schools and the need for such schools to serve the African American communities. However, his work also did not include detail descriptions of the pharmacy programs, nor did it address the challenges the schools faced in trying to remain viable.

Hopefully, this work will add to the topic of African American healthcare providers by focusing on pharmacists. My intent is to raise awareness of the passion that African Americans had for pharmaceutical education and the speed at which they became pharmacists. Because their integration as pharmacists came so soon after being under the bondage of slavery, it was as if though they knew what they could and wanted to achieve, even while being enslaved. To help increase an understanding of their sense of purpose of contributing to the welfare of their own communities, I have tried to introduce some of the first college-educated African American pharmacists in the U.S. However, there is so much more information that is yet to be uncovered, I am almost certain that I may have unintentionally overlooked someone and some event that maybe proclaimed to be the first. I hope that you would share this information with students, fellow pharmacists, and the public, not just as African American history, but as part of American history.

Introduction

In the late nineteenth century and early twentieth century, there were two movements occurring simultaneously in the United States (U.S.) that was having a significant impact on the demographics in the profession of pharmacy. One was the Women's Movement[1] which led to a new influx of women into the pharmacy profession for the first time. The effects of that movement continue today as women now make up most practicing pharmacists and over 60% of the applicants to pharmacy schools. The second was the emergence of college-educated African Americans as pharmacists in less than ten years after the American Civil War. Despite the many challenges that were occurring at the same time, by the beginning of the twentieth century, several hundred college-trained African American pharmacists found themselves working in drug stores, dispensaries, and laboratory facilities throughout the U.S. for the first time.[2] Although there were a number of contributing forces to this change, one that is often overlooked and will be explored in more detail is the contributions of the African American pharmacy schools.

Today, there are seven schools that continue to produce most African American pharmacists in the United States. Howard University is the oldest, which started in 1868 and graduated the first African American and only student (Dr. James T. Wormley) in the pharmacy class of 1870.[3] The other schools include Xavier University of Louisiana College of Pharmacy (1927); Texas Southern University (then Texas State University for Negroes) School of Pharmacy (1948) in Houston, Texas; Florida A&M University School of Pharmacy (1951) in Tallahassee, Florida; Hampton University School of Pharmacy (1997) in Hampton, Virginia; Chicago State University College of Pharmacy (1998) in Chicago, Illinois; and University of Maryland Eastern Shores School of Pharmacy (2010) in Princess Anne, Maryland.

Largely forgotten are those African American pharmacy schools that were formed during the late 19th and early 20th century that are now defunct, but not before graduating a significant number of African American pharmacists into the profession for the first time in the history of the country. Included in this review will be: (1) the

Meharry Pharmaceutical College (Nashville, TN); (2) Shaw Leonard School of Pharmacy (Raleigh, NC); (3) University of West Tennessee College of Pharmacy (Memphis, TN); (4) New Orleans University College of Pharmacy of Flint Medical College (New Orleans, LA); (5) Louisville National Medical College Pharmacy Department (Louisville, KY); and (6) the Frelinghuysen University School of Pharmacy. The school that will not be reviewed at this time is the Washington College of Pharmacy (Washington, DC), which was opened from 1922 to 1926.[4]

Often these schools' history, struggles, and accomplishments are not well-documented and appear less often in the pages of pharmacy history books, therefore, remain relatively untold. In recalling their history, it is the hope that the information presented will raise awareness of their existence, impact, and significance to the pharmacy profession today. This review will focus on: (1) the pharmacy education of African Americans after the American Civil War (1868–1970s); (2) the evolution of pharmacy schools for African Americans; and (3) some of the challenges they faced in an atmosphere of racial hostilities and insurmountable educational reforms.

1 Early Realities

John E. Clark, Deborah E. Williams, Sarah J. Steinhardt

The emergence of African American pharmacists ran parallel with the emergence of African American physicians in medicine. Prior to the Civil War, there were very few African Americans who were college-educated and trained as pharmacists. Approximately four million were slaves, and they had no civil rights or independence to life, liberty, or the pursuit of happiness. Those who were free, who could go to school, were restricted, or prohibited from attending professional degree programs in the U.S. Like some physicians, a small number of African American pharmacists received formal training in Europe and in some Northern schools of pharmacy. However, this was not enough to provide an adequate number of African American healthcare providers to care for African American patients, especially during the healthcare crisis created at the end of the Civil War. From the perspective of the military, the healthcare crisis began during the Civil War with the African American soldiers, where an estimated 95% died of their wounds, diseases, and injuries sustained during the war due to a lack of treatment. After the Civil War and the abolishment of slavery (U.S. Constitution 13th Amendment), African Americans experienced more acute medical problems with much less than the rudimentary medical care that was once received on the plantation. As they migrated to larger cities throughout the South, they became more vulnerable to epidemic diseases and poor sanitary environments due to overcrowded living arrangements, diets, and poverty. Because of the lack of adequate healthcare, the deaths among newly emancipated African Americans was almost twice that of whites from the 1870s into the 1890s.[5]

The Freedman Bureau, which was created when President Abraham Lincoln signed into law the Freedman's Bureau Act on March 3, 1865,[6] intended to aid the former slaves with food and shelter, education, and healthcare. (See **Figure** 1.) It was the government's first effort in providing healthcare services for any group of its citizens.[7] However, the medical services provided were temporary and very insufficient to meet demand. Several fraternal associations, a few doctors, and religious organizations that had advocated for such a Bureau before the law was passed, also provided support and some basic informal medical services. Even with the support of the various religious groups, the medical services were not enough.

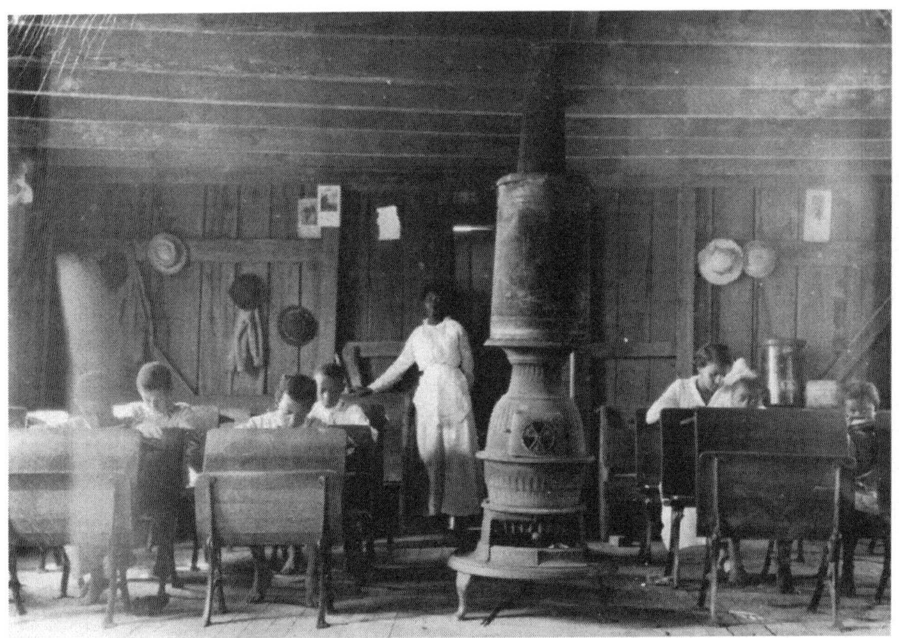

FIGURE 1. Freedom Bureau School.

(Source: Civil Rights Movement in Virginia. "The Beginning of Black Education." Virginia Historical Society, http://www.vahistorical.org/collections-and-resources/virginia-history-explorer/civil-rights-movement-virginia/beginnings-black [accessed January 31, 2018].)

The healthcare crisis was particularly profound in southern states identified as the "black belt,"[8] where the largest concentration of African Americans existed (>50% of the county population) from the 1790s through the 1960s. It was also the area where the need for healthcare was greatest and where there were not enough educated

African American healthcare providers to serve the people who needed it the most. By 1910, it was estimated that 9.8 million African Americans in the south (in the "black belt") were in need of healthcare.[9] Despite the exponential growth in the African American population, southern white medical and pharmacy schools continued to not accept African American students. The American Medical Association (AMA) also endorsed the recommendation of the Carnegie Foundation's Flexner Report to close approximately 40% of U.S. medical colleges.[10] By 1923, 5 out 7 of the African American medical schools, which were established between 1868–1907 for the purpose of serving the African American communities, were forced to close.[11] The decision had a profound impact on African Americans' opportunities for medical education and on the health of their communities. Years later, as the number of African American physicians decreased and lagged far behind the African American population growth,[12] there were not enough African American physicians to meet the healthcare needs of their communities. It has been suggested that the health disparities seen today are the result of the healthcare crisis created at the end of the Civil War and the impact of the closing of the African American medical schools.[13]

Other African American healthcare practitioners were also affected. Four of the medical colleges that were forced to closed also produced dentists, nurses, and pharmacists.[14] As the number of African American physician graduates decreased and became less available to their communities, so did the numbers of dentists, nurses, and pharmacists. The trend showing low numbers of black pharmacists continued for decades. By 1940, it was projected that the number of African American graduating from pharmacy schools had fallen to less than 20 graduates per year following the closing of the Meharry Pharmaceutical College in 1937.[15] By 1947, it was estimated that there was only one African American pharmacist to every 22,815 African American citizens versus one white pharmacist for every 1,714 white citizens in the population. The number of white pharmacists was estimated to be thirteen (13.3) times that of African American pharmacists and that number varied considerably by state, ranging from twice as many in Delaware to 55 times as many in Mississippi.[16]

Actions that promoted the education of African Americans in pharmacy

Over time, several political and social initiatives tended to promote the education and integration of African Americans in pharmacy. Some of those which will not be explored here include:

- Federal legislation prohibiting discrimination based on race and sex in employment and in education,[17]
- Federal legislation creating opportunities for women in education,[18]
- Activism for change in discriminatory practices in education, employment, and in federal regulations,[19]
- Increases in federal funding that encouraged recruitment of more students in colleges of pharmacy,[20]
- Increases in the number of pharmacy schools nationally,[21]
- Professional associations and universities change in philosophy with more focus on diversity, gender, and inclusion.[22]

Early political initiatives that had an indirect impact on the pharmacy education of African Americans may be associated with the Morrill Act of 1862 and the Freedmen's Bureau Act of 1865. The Freedmen's Bureau was headed by Union General Oliver Otis Howard from May 1865 to July 1874. Under General Howard's leadership, the Bureau not only established schools for the nearly four million freed slaves, but also supervised contracts between Freedmen and employers, managed confiscated lands, and provided food, shelter, clothing, and medical care. When Washington, D.C. chartered a new school of higher education for African Americans on March 2, 1867, it was named Howard University in honor of General Oliver O. Howard who served as its president up until 1874. Early on Howard University began awarding degrees in medicine, dentistry, and pharmacy that continues today.[23] The College of Pharmacy evolved from the Pharmaceutical Department within Howard's Medical Department in 1868. It officially became the Pharmaceutical College in 1870 and in

1882 was referred to in the Medical school's catalogue as "The Medical Department comprising the Medical College, the Dental College, and the Pharmaceutical College."[24] The pharmacy school enrollment started very small, with only four students graduating between 1870 and 1881.[25] By 1900, the Pharmaceutical College at Howard University had graduated a total of 108 students. (See **Table 1**.)

TABLE 1. Pharmacy Graduates from Howard University Medical Department: 1868–1900

Session	Students	Graduates
1868–1869	1	—
1869–1870	1	1
1870–1871	1	—
1871–1872	6	1
1872–1873	2	—
1873–1874	—	—
1874–1875	—	—
1875–1876	—	—
1876–1877	—	—
1878–1879	—	—
1879–1880	1	1
1880–1881	1	1
1881–1882	2	—
1882–1883	7	7
1883–1884	4	1
1884–1885	4	2
1885–1886	9	—
1886–1887	17	6
1887–1888	23	13
1888–1889	15	5
1889–1890	5	5
1890–1891	6	1
1891–1892	17	8

Session	Students	Graduates
1892–1893	14	7
1893–1894	19	5
1894–1895	14	6
1895–1896	18	5
1896–1897	17	8
1897–1898	22	7
1898–1899	18	6
1899–1900	26	12
Total	**270**	**108**

Source: David Smith Lamb. "*Howard University Medical Department: A Historical, Biographical and Statistical Souvenir.*" (Washington, D.C.: Beresford, 1900), 143. (-) indicates no data reported.

The Freedmen Hospital, which was established in 1862 in the District of Columbia (D.C.) to care for the freed and sick African Americans, became the primary teaching hospital for the Howard University Medical School. The pharmacy dispensary located within the hospital also became one of the early hospital pharmacy practice sites for graduates and students of the Howard University Pharmaceutical College. *Julia Pearl Hughes'* training as a Howard University pharmacy student in the Freedman Hospital, led to her being employed as one of the first African American females to be in charge of a hospital pharmacy, when she accepted a position at the Frederick Douglas Memorial Hospital (Philadelphia, PA) after graduation in 1897. In 1900, she left the hospital to open Hughes Pharmacy in Philadelphia, making her, what some believe, to be the first African American female to own a drugstore in America.[26]

Before the Civil War ended, President Abraham Lincoln had signed into law the Morrill Act of 1862.[27] The Act provided states with federal funding for higher education by granting them federally controlled land to sell for raising funds to establish endowments to teach and award degrees related to agriculture, the mechanic arts, and later engineering, and Reserve Officers' Training Programs (ROTC). Based on provisions in the law, the more populous eastern states benefitted the most from the Act because they received more land than less populous states. The confederate states of the south were excluded because the ongoing Civil War was considered an act to overthrow the government, which was one of the criteria in the bill for disqualification. The government left it up to each state to come up with the details on how they would execute the law under its provisions and requirements. Because most states embraced the *"separate but equal"* doctrine[28] contained in the bill, it had a profound negative impact on the educational opportunities for African Americans. As a result, 17 states excluded African Americans from access to the land grant colleges without providing equal education as was mandated in the bill.[29]

The Morrill Act of 1862 was later extended in 1890 and became known as the Morrill Land Grant College Act.[30] The amended law provided cash rather land, and included the former confederate states of the South, but with unfavorable provisions for funding that race not be included in the criteria for admission of students in the colleges. In response to the provision, while still embracing the separate but equal doctrine, the states set up separate land grand colleges for the education of African Americans. This change accelerated the number of pharmacy programs in the land grant colleges and universities and the development of separate pharmacy programs for African Americans in the historically black colleges and universities (HBCUs).[31]

Although most black schools are referred to as HBCUs, not all were initiated from land or grants under the Morrill Land Grant College Act. None of the early defunct African American pharmacy schools benefited from the Morrill Land Grant College Act. Most were started with no grants or land from the state and often evolved with the purchase of various free-standing buildings where classes were held. All were supported with private funding, or supported by various religious organizations, which included the Freedmen's Aid Society of the Methodist Episcopal Church,[32] the American Baptist Home Mission Society, and the American Missionary Association.[33] The major religious organizations also sought to address the medical and economic crisis by educating former slaves in literacy, basic knowledge of reading and writing, religion, and practical job and domestic skills. Some of the schools also developed programs that offered degrees in medicine, dentistry, nursing, and pharmacy. The intent was to create schools that would train competent black health care providers to treat and take care of the medical needs of the black communities, which were being provided substandard and unequal healthcare and were systematically excluded by the current "health system."

Nine pharmacy schools for African Americans opened between 1868 and 1927. (See **Table 2**.) By 1937, seven of the schools had closed for several reasons, but mainly because of financial constraints in trying to keep up with changing educational standards and racism.[34]

TABLE 2. Pharmacy Schools that Trained Most African Americans

Name	Location	Year Opened	Year Closed	Affiliation
Howard University College of Pharmacy	Washington, DC	1868	Active	Independent
Meharry Pharmaceutical College	Nashville, TN	1890	1937	Freedmen's Aid Society of the Methodist Episcopal Church
Shaw Leonard School of Pharmacy	Raleigh, NC	1890	1918	American Baptist Mission Society
University of West Tennessee Department of Pharmacy	Jackson, TN *(1900–1907)*; Memphis, TN *(1907–1923)*	1900	1923	Independent, proprietary
New Orleans University College of Pharmacy of Flint Medical College	New Orleans, LA	1900	1915	Freedmen's Aid Society of the Methodist Episcopal Church
Louisville National Medical College Department of Pharmacy	Louisville, KY	1902	1912	Independent, proprietary

Frelinghuysen University School of Pharmacy	Washington, DC	1917	1927	Independent, proprietary
Washington College of Pharmacy	Washington, D.C.	1922	1926	Independent, proprietary
Xavier University of New Orleans College of Pharmacy	New Orleans, LA	1927	Active	Sisters of the Blessed Sacrament
Texas Southern University College of Pharmacy	Houston, TX	1948	Active	Independent Public
Florida A&M University College of Pharmacy	Tallahassee, FL	1951	Active	Public
Hampton University School of Pharmacy	Hampton, VA	1997	Active	Private
Chicago State University College of Pharmacy	Chicago, IL	1998	Active	Public
University of Maryland Eastern Shore School of Pharmacy	Princess Anne, M.D.	2010	Active	Public

Source: *"1879-1907 Twenty-eighth Annual Announcement of State University and 1888-1907 Twentieth Announcement of Louisville National Medical College, 1907-1908,* (Louisville, KY: Louisville National Medical College, 1908); Todd Lee Savitt, "Four African-American Proprietary Medical Colleges: 1882-1923." *Journal of the History of Medicine and Allied Sciences,* 55.3(July 2000): 206-207.

Post-Slavery Reactions to African Americans

As the country grappled with the black health dilemma, the issues of civil rights and racism intensified. The educational accomplishments of the early African American healthcare providers, regardless of their occupational status, were not enough to protect them from the effects of the racism and civil rights violations. While the government had tried to integrate and protect all African Americans into society, its laws too were ineffective in curtailing the racism. The Civil Rights Act of 1866[35] was to affirm the citizenship of person of African descent born or brought into the country and was intended to protect the civil rights of those individuals. The law also provided support for African Americans to vote in elections for the first time. Because of the ineffectiveness of the law, the Civil Rights Act of 1875[36] was passed with provisions to address discrimination involving public accommodations, public transportation, and jury participation. In 1883, the U.S. Supreme Court nullified the Civil Rights Act of 1875, declaring certain sections of the law to be unconstitutional.[37] In a sense, this action left African Americans with no protection regarding their civil and legal rights. On May 18, 1896, the Supreme Court rendered a decision in the case of *Plessy vs Ferguson*[38] that upheld the constitutionality of state-mandated laws requiring racial segregation under the doctrine of "*separate but equal.*"[39] By the beginning of the 20th century, all former Confederate states had restricted the civil rights and civil liberties of African Americans by strictly and violently enforcing racial segregation for decades under what became known as the "Jim Crow" laws.[40] Lynching and public burnings increased in numbers with over 3,400 African American men and women lynched between 1889 and 1922, sometimes for frivolous complaints, and 28 publicly burned to death between 1918 to 1921 with very rare prosecutions for the events.[41] African Americans were not only barred from hotels, restaurants, public housing, amusement parks and beaches, but were also restricted in employment, in using public transportation, medical facilities, and in attending some educational institutions.

Public Reactions Involving African American Pharmacists

Although educated and sometimes prosperous, African American pharmacists were mistreated the same as other African American citizens. On May 25, 1918, pharmacist *Julia Pearl Hughes Coleman*, then President of the Hair-Vim Chemical Company, was physically forced to give up her first-class seat while traveling from Baltimore to Washington, DC, aboard the Baltimore and Annapolis Electric Railway. (See **Figure** 2.) In her determination to change the discriminatory practices, she filed a lawsuit against the railway. The judge ruled in her favor. However, her case like many others was trivialized by the courts in awarding just $20.00 for damages but did not change the law or the practice.[42]

JimCrowed

Dr. Julia P. H. Coleman president of the Hair-Vim Chemical Company was recently awarded a judgement against the Washington, Baltimore and Annapolis Interurban line, successfully sustaining a charge that she was "Jimcrowed" during a trip from Baltimore to Washington, in violation of her constitutional rights as an interstate passenger. A mass of complaints are being made against electric line and it is likely that suits will reach the United States Supreme Court before the corporation can be compelled to quit its daily violation of the laws relating to interstate travel. Source: *Nashville Globe, July 26, 1918, p. 3*

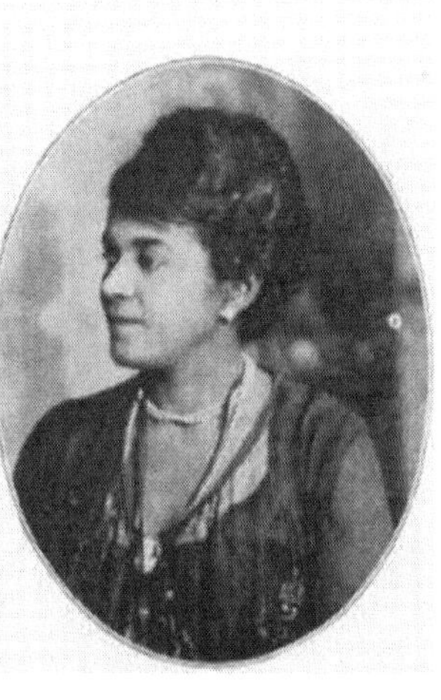

FIGURE 2. Julia Pearl Hughes, Jim Crowed.

In a similar experience while using public transportation in 1950, pharmacist *Gwendolyn Wilson Fowler* sued the popular Rock Island Railroad for discriminating against her when traveling aboard the train between Des Moines, Iowa, and Kansas City, Missouri. The employees of the train seated her in a non-segregated dining car but put a curtain around her table so that she would be separated from other white passengers. She was also moved to a segregated area ("Jim Crow section") of the train by employees when promised a sleeper car by the conductor.[43] Her suit, again, did not change the practice.

The trend carried over into the military where African American pharmacists serving as soldiers in the Army were subjected to the same mistreatment. Captain *Matthew Virgil Boutte*, a registered pharmacist of African and French descent, was placed under military arrest for interacting with the French speaking citizen and later court-martialed for not abiding by the American "Jim Crow" laws while serving in France during World War I.[44] To avoid a wrongful, dishonorable discharge, he hired a skillful attorney and became one of the lucky ones who won his case in court and went on to become a very successful pharmacist in New York.[45] (See **Figure 3**.)

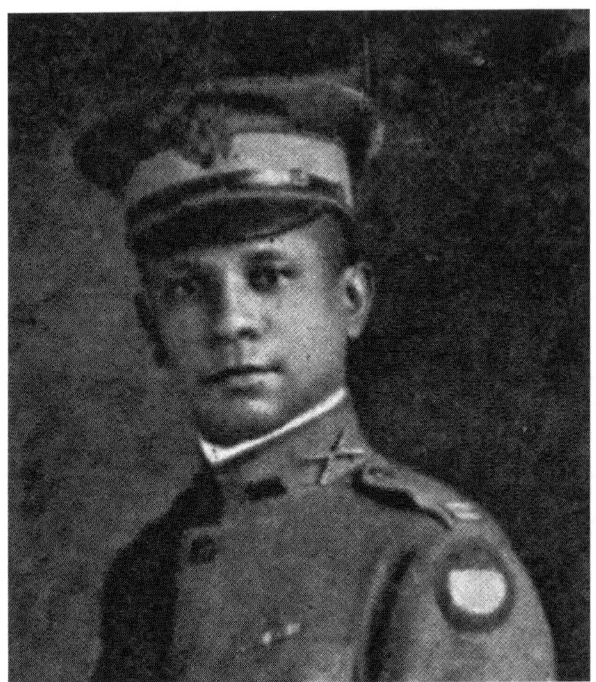

FIGURE 3. Captain Matthew Virgil Boutte.

(Source: Addie W. Hunton and Kathryn M. Johnson, *Two Colored Women With the American Expeditionary Forces*. Brooklyn, NY: Brooklyn Eagle Press, 1920, pp. 57-61.)

Zirl A. Palmer, an African American pharmacist from Lexington, Kentucky, was not permitted to play in the May 1958 Kentucky State Closed Tennis Championships after advancing and becoming one of the top seeded, state-ranked competitive tennis players. (See **Figure 4**.) The Kentucky State Tennis Association declared his upcoming match with Henry Baughman a loss by default because the Idle Hour Golf Club that owned the tennis courts barred African Americans from participating in activities on their properties. Palmer did not protest the decision and therefore could not advance in the competition.[46] On September 5, 1968, Zirl A. Palmer was involved in another unfortunate incident when the drugstore he owned was demolished by a bomb placed in the store by a former Ku Klux Klan member, who was upset over Palmer's business success, advocacy and leadership involving matters of civil rights in the community of Lexington. (See **Figure 5**.) Injured in the blast along with Palmer was his wife Marian, and their four-year-old daughter, Andrea.[47] After Palmer and his family recovered from the incident, he continued to work as a pharmacist, but did not re-open his drugstore. In 1972, he later became the first African American to be appointed to the University of Kentucky Board of Trustees.[48]

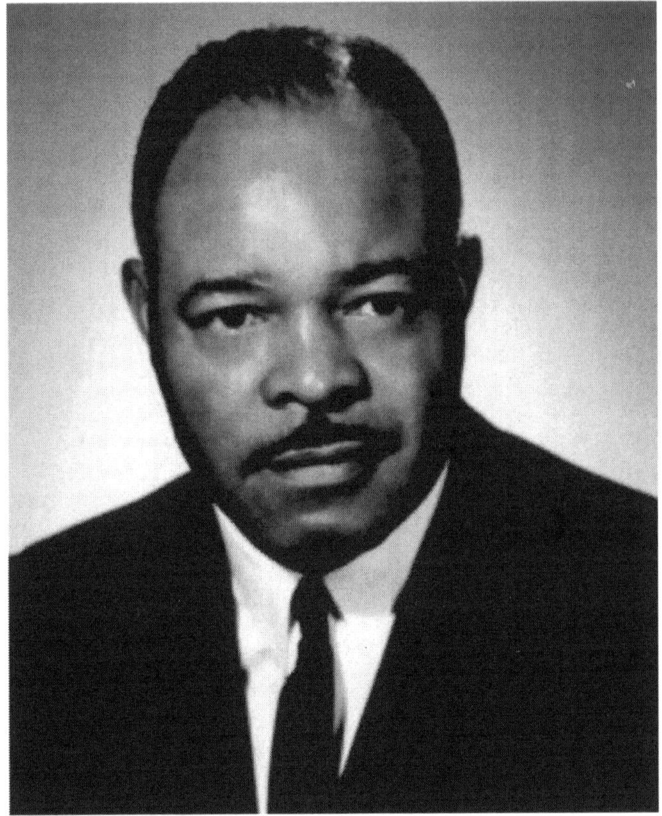

FIGURE 4. Zirl A. Palmer.

(Source: *Kentucky Yearbook*, 1972)

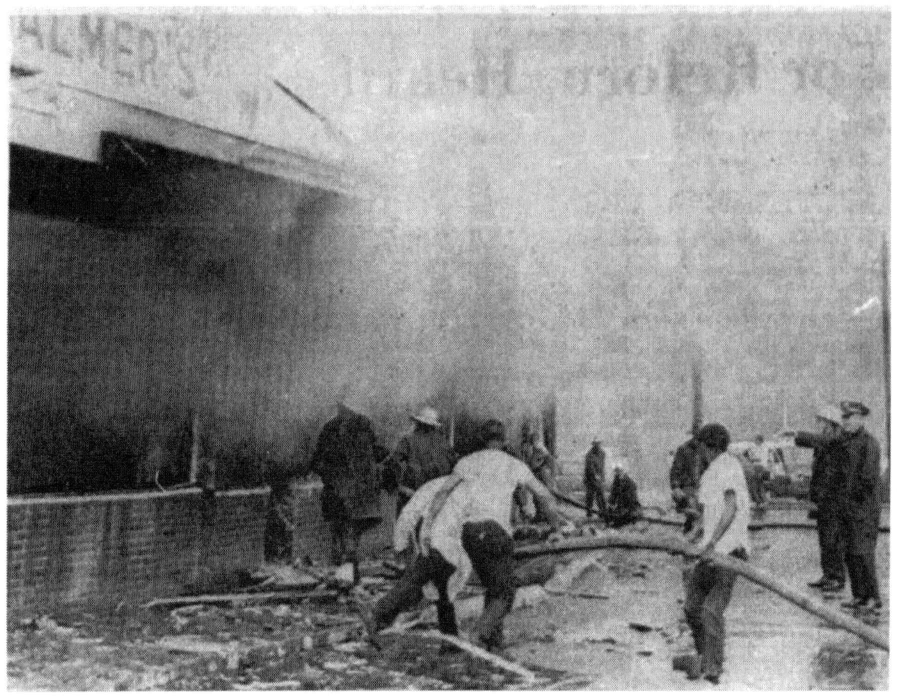

FIGURE 5. "Blast Injures Store Occupants."

(Source: *Courier Journal*, September 5, 1968, 49.)

Reactions to African American Pharmacists by Other Pharmacists

The emergence of African Americans into the pharmacy profession was not without reactions from other pharmacists. Before 1900, the total number of African American pharmacists in the U.S. was estimated to be approximately 65.[49] By 1932, the numbers were estimated to have increased to 330, with 80 African American pharmacists in Northern states and 250 African American pharmacists in Southern states.[50] From 1940 to 1950, the percentage of African American pharmacists to all pharmacists was estimated to be 1.1 and 1.6 percent, respectively. Although small in numbers, their presence was felt and created attention throughout the profession.[51] Like women integrating pharmacy for the first time, there was significant opposition, stereotypes, and questions from other pharmacists and the public.[52]

Some white pharmacists questioned if it was right to hire African American pharmacists in their drugstores.[53] African American pharmacists were often not allowed to work in some white owned drugstores, to obtain apprenticeships, or pharmacy practice experiences because of concerns by the owners that their presence would be detrimental to their business and reduce their profits.[54] Proprietors and the public also seemed to doubt their ability to practice as pharmacists, their education and training, and their ability to learn and know the drugstore business.[55] Attitudes towards working with black pharmacists continued in some area into the 1960s (see Reflection).

As some African Americans began to open their own drugstores, it was not uncommon for white pharmacists to not patronize or collaborate with black drugstore owners or black patients who brought them prescriptions.[56] While some white pharmacists would fill the prescriptions of black patients, they would prohibit the patients from using their popular lunch counters and soda fountains and, in some cases, the patients would be prohibited from entering their drugstores.[57]

Many questions about African American pharmacists also came from African American patients and physicians who would not patronize the African American-owned drugstores, but instead preferred to take their business to white drugstores.[58] In addition, some African American physicians became drugstore owners and were more successful than independent African American pharmacists. Because they were physicians, they had more financial capital and suppliers were more likely to extend credit. This meant their stores were often better stocked with pharmaceuticals, organized and clean, and they had the trust of the African American community.[59] The lack of community trust by African American patients, together with challenges in maintaining well-stocked, clean and organized drugstores that were competitive and comparable to white drugstores, created more difficulties for African Americans to make a living as independent pharmacists.[60] Such challenges not only led to differences between white and black pharmacists in employment opportunities, income and salaries, ownership of drugstores, they also affected the pharmaceutical services provided in their communities and the occupational outlook for African Americans as pharmacists.[61]

Other factors that affected opportunities for African American pharmacists included the nature of the pharmacy business and the expansion of commercial chain drugstores. Historically, family owned pharmacy businesses were kept in the family. They employed family members and rarely hired African Americans as pharmacists. After World War II, commercial chain drugstores started moving their businesses to the suburbs along with the flight of people from the urban cities. The pharmacists employed in the stores would include those who lived in the suburbs, which commonly were not African Americans.[62] A survey published by Meharry Medical College in 1932 found that 20% of African American pharmacy graduates never started their careers or practices as pharmacists.[63] It is unclear whether some did not see a future in pharmacy or had occupational difficulties trying to start their careers.

Reactions to African Americans in the Pharmacy Schools

Northern Schools. Prior to and after the Civil War, many pharmacy schools of higher education would not admit African American students. Some schools in the North would do so, but in very small deliberate numbers. Pharmacy schools that accepted some of the first African Americans in the late nineteenth and early twentieth centuries (see **Appendix A**) included:

- **College of Pharmacy of the City of New York** (later became Columbia University)
    - 1844 – *Phillip A. White*, pharmacy diploma given.[64]
    - 1850 – *Peter W. Ray*, pharmacy diploma given.[65]
    - 1895 – *Frank L. Chambers*, Ph.G. conferred.[66]
    - 1919 – *Robinson M. Haden*, Ph.G. conferred.[67]
    - 1923 – *Etnah Rochon Boutte, Cyrus T.L. Dabney, Joseph Jennings, Otho Gather Harbison, Elwood Melrose Osborne, Wallace Stewart Hayes,* Ph.G. conferred.[68]
    - 1927 – *Lillian Smith, Vera Irvin, Artrelle Levy*, Ph.G. conferred.[69]

- **University of Illinois College of Pharmacy**
  - 1891 – *John Meade Benson*, Ph.G. conferred.[70]
  - 1911 – *Solomon Leroy Lee,* Ph.G.; *Matthew Virgil Boutte*, Ph.G., Ph.C. conferred.[71]
  - 1912 – *William Sylvester White*, Ph.G. conferred.[72]
- **University of Michigan School of Pharmacy**
  - 1892 – *George R. Jackson*, Ph.C. conferred. He was the first black pharmacist in Memphis, Tennessee.[73]
  - 1907 – *Edgar Burnett Keemer*, Ph.C. conferred.[74]
  - 1908 – *Augustus Alphonza Williams*, Ph.C., B.S.
  - 1910 – *Nicholas Alfred Garfield Diggs*, Ph.C., *Norris Augustus Dodson,* Ph.C. (1908), B.S. conferred.[75]
  - 1912 – *Ewell E. Clemons,* Ph.C.; *James H. Hilburn,* Ph.C. conferred
  - 1913 – *Basie S. Braxton*, Ph.C. conferred
  - 1914 – *Curtis F. Jenkins*, Ph.C.; *Max W. Johnson*, Ph.C. conferred
  - 1923 – *Ernest Linwood Harris*, Ph.C., B.S. conferred.[76]
- **Philadelphia College of Pharmacy** (today the University of the Sciences in Philadelphia)
  - 1895 – *Henry McKee Minton*, Ph.G. conferred; who went on to become the co-founder and first superintendent of Mercy Hospital in Philadelphia, PA (later merged and became Mercy-Douglas Hospital). [77]
  - 1899 – *John Allen McFall*, Ph.G. conferred
  - 1917 – *Maurice B. Dabney*, Ph.G., Ph.C. conferred.[78]
  - 1923 – *Effie Nevers*, Ph.G. conferred.
- **New Jersey College of Pharmacy** (now Rutgers Ernest Mario School of Pharmacy)

- 1898 – *Charles Bernardo*, Ph.G. conferred.[79]
- 1923 – *Alice M. Bunce, Edgar D. Giggetts*, ph.G. conferred.[80]

- **Brooklyn College of Pharmacy** (today Arnold & Marie Schwartz College of Pharmacy)
  - 1892 – *Joseph Francis Smith,* Ph.G. conferred.[81]
  - 1895 – *William H. Smith, Jr*., Ph.G. conferred.[82]
  - 1908 – *Anna Louise James,* Ph.G. conferred,[83] making her one of the first African American females to receive a pharmacy degree from a predominantly white institution and the first to be licensed as a pharmacist in the state of Connecticut.
  - 1923 – *Archie A. Miller*, Ph.G. conferred.[84]
  - 1927 – *Charles Herbert Gurley*, Ph.G.
- **Highland Park College, Department of Pharmacy** (merged and today Drake University College of Pharmacy)
  - 1906 – *William Joseph Waters*, Ph.G.
  - 1908 – *Hattie Hutchinson*, awarded the Ph.G.,[85] making her one of the first African American females to receive a pharmacy degree from a predominantly white institution and the first to become licensed as a pharmacist in the state of Iowa.
- **Temple University College of Pharmacy**
  - 1911 – *Ruth Gardena Birnie, Camille O. Green-Mims*, Ph.G. awarded.[86]
  - 1916 – *Walter Lee Brandon, Raymond H. Rodgers*, Ph.G. conferred.[87]
  - 1919 – *William M. Banner, Percival L. Bedward, Anna P. Comegys, Norman L. Glenn, Edward Howell, Percival L. Martin*, Ph.G. conferred.[88]

- 1920 – *Romanus M. Fields, Philippe Dartiguenave, Gelia V. Harris, Oley E. Horsey, George T. Hunter, Benjamin Williams,* Ph.G. conferred.
- 1922 – *E. Bennett, W. N. Bowser, G. C. Brown, M. N. Gibbs, C. L. Holland, P. L. Martin, J. H. Patterson, S. L. Scott, W. H. Wormley*, Ph.G. conferred.[89]
- 1923 – *Albre R. Artice, Mary E. Brown, Spurgeon D. Brown, Raymond Bounds, Archer A. Clayton, Horace Clinton, Edith R. Green, Herbert R. Hamill, Susie Hampton, Eva G. Hall, Alvin S. Hawkes, Marjorie Smith, Mabel S. Manigault, Mary H. Moore, William A. McGuire, Thomas J. Potter, Josiah Robinson, Cleophus Shaw, George Tilghman,* Ph.G. conferred.[90]
- 1926 – *Rosa Alexander, Theodore Brown, William Dean, Ruth Downing, Paul M. Foster, Audrey Gray, John H. Loper, Frances Moses, Benjamin Warner, Quincy Waters, Maris Wesley, George M. White, John F. Williams, Joseph M. Williams, Henry H. Winters*, Ph.G. conferred.[91]

- **University of Washington College of Pharmacy**
  - 1912 – *Alice Augusta Ball,* Ph.C. (1912), B.S. (Bachelor of Science, 1914) awarded.[92]
  - 1916 – *Lodie M. Biggs*, Ph.C. (1916), B.S. (1921) conferred.[93]
- **University of Minnesota College of Pharmacy**
  - 1911 – *James Louis Titus*, Ph.B. (Bachelor of Pharmacy) conferred.[94]
  - 1913 – *Raymond W. Cannon*, Ph.B. conferred.[95]
  - 1915 – *Olive D. Howard (Crosthwait),* Ph.B. conferred.[96]
  - 1916 – *Miles O. Cannon*, Ph.G. conferred.[97]
  - 1923 – *George King, Hutchins F. Inge, Frederick D. Inge,* Ph.G. conferred.

  - 1927 – *Chauncey I. Cooper*, Ph.C.
- **University of Pittsburgh College of Pharmacy**
  - 1914 – *Wesley Rollo Wilson, William Wyatt Stewart, Henry David Primas*, Ph.G. conferred.[98]
  - 1915 – *Stanley Wilbert Jefferson*, Ph.G. conferred
  - 1916 – *Ella Phillips Stewart* (then Ella Phillips Myers), Ph.G. conferred; making her the first African American female to receive a pharmacy degree from the school; *Richard B. Carter, George G. Williams,* Ph.G. awarded; *Charlotte Louisa Austin,* awarded Certificate of Proficiency (Maderia Medica).[99]
  - 1921 – *William L. Manggrum*, Ph.G.
- **University of Wisconsin School of Pharmacy**
  - 1920 – *Leo V. Butts,* Ph.G. conferred.[100] First African American to graduate from the UW School of Pharmacy.
- **University of Iowa College of Pharmacy**
  - 1907 – *Edward William Thompson*, Ph.G. conferred.[101]
  - 1909 – *George O. Caldwell, St. Julien Doyle Drayton*, Ph.G. conferred.[102]
  - 1921 – *Lorena Suggs*, Ph.G. conferred.[103]
- **University of Kansas School of Pharmacy**
  - 1897 – *Spurgeon Nathaniel Gray*, Ph.C.
  - 1917 – *Ada Pearl Bell,* Ph.C., Ph.G.
- **Ohio State University College of Pharmacy**
  - 1897 – *Arthur K. Lawrence*, Ph.G.[104]
  - 1913 – *Fannie C. Jamison, Florence Maye Burns*, Ph.G. conferred.[105]

- 1921 – *Howard Swayne Lindsay,* Ph.G. conferred; *Spotwood McKinley Greene,* Ph.C. conferred.[106]

- **Massachusetts College of Pharmacy**
  - 1904 – *Charles Henry Horton*, Ph.B. awarded.[107]
  - 1914 – *Bertran F. Jones,* Ph.G.[108]
  - 1915 – *Rosamond Alice Guinn,* Ph.G.[109]
  - 1921 – *Antoine E. Green,* Ph.B. awarded;[110] *Mary B. Hill,* Ph.G.[111]
- **Case Western Reserve University College of Pharmacy**
  - 1923 – *Robert Harris Shauter*, Ph.C. conferred.[112]
- **University of Buffalo College of Pharmacy**
  - 1916 – *Cyrus F. Dozier*, Ph.B. awarded.[113]
- **College of the City of Detroit School of Pharmacy** (later became Wayne State University)
  - 1927 – *Muriel I. Dorsay,* Ph.C.[114]
  - 1928 – *Pansy A. Stewart*, Ph.C., *Sidney Barthwell,* Ph.C.[115]
  - 1930 – *Thomas T. Matthews*, Ph.C.[116]
  - 1932 – *William Wade Venable*, Ph. C.[117]
- **St. Louis College of Pharmacy**
  - 1897 – *Ernest L. Harris*, Ph.G.
  - 1957 – *Doris Bryson*, *Ve Ella Graham, Margaret Brown*, awarded B.S.
  - 1962 – *George Mitchell, Jr*. B.S.
- **Purdue University College of Pharmacy**
  - 1890 – *George Washington Lacey*, Ph.G.
  - 1923 – *W.F. Jones*, Ph.G. conferred.
  - 1924 – *Olfred (Ova) Oliver Nash,* Ph.G. conferred.

Not all the Northern pharmacy schools admitted African American students without opposition. One of the early reports of racial discrimination in pharmaceutical education occurred in 1883 in Washington, D.C., when the National College of Pharmacy admitted an African American student named *Oliver M. Atwood.* When students learned of the decision, thirty-eight white students, under the leadership of the president of the student pharmacy association, walked out of class in protest; refusing to be in the same class with him.[118] The incident received national attention. Rather than take strong decisive action to prevent such discriminatory behavior, the school conceded to the demands of the opposing students.[119] Oliver Atwood left National and enrolled in the Pharmaceutical College at nearby Howard University, where he was able to continue his educational pursuits in pharmacy and later in medicine. He is listed in the Howard *Alumni Catalogue (1867-1896)* as having received both the Phar.D. and the M.D. degrees.[120]

Similar reactions to African American students attending Highland Park College (Des Moines, IA) led to the barring of all African American admissions to the school. *Hattie Hutchinson* entered Highland Park College Department of Pharmacy in 1906 amidst intense racial tensions. Upon receiving the Graduate in Pharmacy (Ph.G.) degree in 1908, she became the first African American female to earn a pharmacy degree in the state of Iowa and one of the last African Americans to attend the pharmacy program at Highland Park College.[121] Because white students opposed attending classes with black students, in 1908 the school's administration barred all black students from attending Highland Park College.[122] Those seeking admission to the school were outraged by the decision and African American students currently enrolled had to curtail their education and transfer to another school.[123] In 1921, Highland Park College of Pharmacy merged with Des Moines College of Pharmacy, which later became Drake University College of Pharmacy as we know it today.[124]

Ella Nora Phillips Stewart (then Ella P. Myers) was denied admission in her first attempt to enter the University of Pittsburgh College of Pharmacy in 1913.[125] Determined to become a pharmacist, she reapplied, was later admitted in 1914 and graduated with the Ph.G. degree in 1916. The environment in her classes was described in a 2010 report as being very segregated. In the report, it states that white males sat in the first rows of seats in the classes, and were followed, in descending order, by white females, then Jews, and then blacks.[126] When she graduated in 1916, Ella Phillips Stewart became the first African American female to earn a pharmacy degree from the University of Pittsburgh College of Pharmacy. However, she was not alone. Her classmate, *Charlotte L Austin*, received the Certificate of Proficiency (Maderia Media) and *Richard B. Carter* and *George G. Williams,* two African American men in the same class, were also awarded the Ph.G. degree in 1916.[127] Prior to their graduation, there were three African American men in the 1914 class: *Wesley Rollo Wilson, William Wyatt Stewart, and Henry David Primas* and one in the 1915 class: *Stanley Wilbert Jefferson*, who were also awarded the Ph.G. degree.[128]

University of Maryland School of Pharmacy is one of the oldest pharmacy schools in the nation. Chartered in 1841 as the Maryland College of Pharmacy,[129] it was very slow to admit African American students into its programs. In May 1948, *Martin B. Booth*, a 21-year-old man, was the first African American to apply for admission in the School of Pharmacy. A short time later, he received notice that his application had been denied on the grounds that the admission quota had been met for the current class size. A second application submitted by Mr. Booth a few months later was not acted upon because the school term had started and the application process had ended. In September 1948, he filed a lawsuit against the University of Maryland contending that the School of Pharmacy had not admitted him because of his race.[130] The university denied the allegation and issued a public policy statement by the President that all applicants to graduate level and professional degree programs of the University of Maryland are considered for admission on the basis of their qualification regardless of race, creed, or color.[131] After long court delays in deciding the case, Martin Booth was not admitted into the School of Pharmacy despite tremendous support from the Baltimore community, judges and lawyers, and a number of advocacy groups and organizations.[132]He suspended his efforts in trying to attend the University of Maryland and entered Morgan State College (today Morgan State University), where he received a Bachelor of Science degree in 1950.[133] Shortly thereafter, he entered Howard University College of Medicine and graduated with the Doctor of

Medicine (M.D.) degree in 1955.[134] For many years, he was a prominent Adolescent & Pediatric Psychiatrist in the District of Columbia and served as Assistant Professor of Medicine at Howard University College of Medicine.[135]

While the Martin B. Booth case was still pending in court, lawsuits were filed in July 1949 by the legal team of the National Association for the Advancement of Colored People (NAACP) on behalf of six more African American residents of Maryland to gain admission to the University of Maryland.[136] The lawsuits alleged that the students' applications were rejected because of race. *Richard Tyson* was one of the students who sued the university because his application for admission to the School of Pharmacy was also rejected.[137] The 20-year-old student claimed that the university's failure to act on his application was a violation of the Federal Constitution and Supreme Court decisions and asked the City Courts to require the University of Maryland to accept and admit him into the School of Pharmacy. The Court did not rule in his favor, and Richard Tyson was not accepted into the University of Maryland School of Pharmacy. It would be about six years later (1957) before the first African American student would be accepted into the University of Maryland School of Pharmacy.[138]

Southern Schools. For decades, all the predominantly white pharmacy schools in the South were reluctant to admit African American students. By 1947, only 45 of the 65 pharmacy schools in the U.S. admitted African American students and the 20 schools that did not were all located in the South.[139] All the schools based their denial on state mandated laws (aka "Jim Crow" laws) which allowed separate education for African Americans and white Americans, even when they lived in the same states and paid the same taxes. The laws were based on the doctrine of *separate but equal*,[140] while a number of reports had put forth valid arguments that, in no state in which separate schools are legally mandatory, did African Americans receive equal educational opportunities.[141] For more than 20 years, the NAACP legal team sought to end segregation in higher education by challenging the constitutionality of state laws requiring separate schools for its tax-paying citizens. The first court case in the country that challenged the state-mandated laws which allowed for the discrimination against African Americans in higher education was filed in March 1933.[142]

Thomas R. Hocutt, a 24-year-old African American, applied for admission to the University of North Carolina School of Pharmacy. He had the qualifications for admission but was denied by the Dean of Admissions. The basis of the denial was on the grounds that his application did not contain the required documentation set forth by the school's rules and regulations, pertaining to a complete scholastic history, and other information which would support his eligibility for registration and admission.[143] Thomas Hocutt secured the legal counsel of Conrad Pearson and C. Aubrey McCoy of the NAACP and filed a *writ of mandamus* with the state court compelling the University to admit him into the School of Pharmacy.[144] The court ruled in favor of the University of North Carolina citing that Mr. Hocutt had failed to comply with the University's rules and processes required in the application for admission.[145]

A second similar case was filed in 1937 by the NAACP when *William B. Redmond II* sued the University of Tennessee after being denied admission into the School of Pharmacy.[146] In the law suit, Mr. Redmond contended that the state constitutional provision forbidding African Americans attendance at white universities was in direct conflict with the 14th Amendment of the United States Constitution. Because of the conflict, the proposed remedy was that the university should enroll Mr. Redmond in the School of Pharmacy or provide him separate educational accommodations.[147] In April 1937, the Chancery Court judge, Louis D. Bejach, denied the petition of William Redmond to enter the University of Tennessee School of Pharmacy on the grounds that his constitutional rights were not denied and, and stated that if they were, he could have exercised the right to appeal to the Board of Education or to the state legislature (but not to the courts).[148] In an effort that resulted in maintaining the discriminatory practices and separate pharmacy educational opportunities for African Americans, the Tennessee state legislature approved scholarships and grants in the limited amount of $2,500 per person to African American students who wished to pursue a pharmacy education at other programs outside the state of Tennessee.[149]

Although the NAACP did not receive the verdict it sought in the case involving William Redmond and the University of Tennessee, the organization was successful in increasing professional education opportunities for African Americans in other cases. After several delays and almost twenty years later, the court ruled in Thomas Hocutt's favor for admission to the University of North Carolina in 1951.[150] Before the court decision, Thomas Hocutt moved to New York and worked for the NYC Transit Authority. He died in 1974 and never realized his dream of becoming a pharmacist.[151] However, it's generally accepted that the Hocutt case provided the framework for several other cases that broke down barriers to admission at southern universities.[152] From the 1930s thru the 1950s, the NAACP won eleven cases that resulted in Southern state universities either relaxing or removing their policy that banned African American students from being admitted into their professional degree programs (e.g., law, medicine, pharmacy, nursing, engineering, dentistry).[153] Some of the states involved in the court cases included, Louisiana, Texas, Alabama, Georgia, Mississippi, South Carolina, Missouri, Oklahoma, Arkansas, Virginia, West Virginia, Kentucky, and Tennessee.[154]The changes in admission practices led to African American students being admitted to some professional degree programs for the first time and increased equal opportunities for education for all African Americans. Although not all completed the pharmacy program, the following is an incomplete list of some of the first African Americans admitted to schools in the South (see **Appendix B**) following desegregation:

- **University of North Carolina College of Pharmacy** – *William Wicker*, first to integrate the College of Pharmacy, attended 1962-1965;[155] *Mona Yvonne Boston*, awarded the B.S. degree in 1967, the first African American female to graduate.[156]
- **University of Mississippi School of Pharmacy** – *George Leonard,* awarded the B.S. degree, 1969;[157] *Theron Evans* admitted in 1970, but transferred to Texas Southern University School of Pharmacy after one year;[158] *Clarence Earl Dubose*, awarded the B.S. degree, 1975;[159] *Harold B. Blakley,* awarded the B.S. degree, 1976;[160] *Jacqueline K. Henderson,* first African American female admitted in 1973;[161] *Gloria Jean Rush*, attended 1974;[162] *Wendall Leonard,* attended 1975.[163]

- **Medical University of South Carolina College of Pharmacy** – *James L. Hodges,* first African American to integrate the College of Pharmacy; awarded the B.S. degree in 1971.[164]
- **Samford University School of Pharmacy** – *Arthur Radcliff,* attended 1971;[165] *Harold Boggarty, Ronald V. Jones,* attended 1972;[166] *Theotus Butler* awarded the B.S. degree, 1973.[167]
- **Auburn University School of Pharmacy** – *Phyllis Washington Gosa* awarded B.S. degree, 1974. She was the first African American female graduate from the School of Pharmacy;[168] *Linwood Moore* awarded B.S. degree, 1977.[169]
- **University of Georgia School of Pharmacy** – *William Robie* attended 1969-1970;[170] *Richard Morgan* (1971-1974) B.S., *Alonzo Wilson* attended 1971;[171] *Willie Reed* attended 1972;[172] *Patricia Ann Palms* attended 1973-1978, B.S.;[173]
- **University of Kentucky College of Pharmacy** – *William R. Schultz* attended 1953-1954.[174]
- **University of Tennessee College of Pharmacy** – *James Saarnell Hayes*, first African American to earn his B.S. in Pharmacy degree (1973); and the first to earn the Doctor of Pharmacy (Pharm.D.) degree (1974).[175]
- **University of Arkansas for Medical Sciences – School of Pharmacy** – *Carl Brooks,* B.S. (1957);[176] *Marion K. Greene,* attended Junior year, 1961.[177]
- **University of Florida College of Pharmacy** – *Ira Charles Robinson,* B.S. (FAMU), Ph.D. (UF), 1966.
- **Mercer's Southern School of Pharmacy**
    - 1967 – *Ronald Myrick,* B.S.
    - 1968 – *Hewitt Matthews,* B.S.

In 1947, the only two HBCU pharmacy schools that remained open were the Howard University and Xavier University of Louisiana Colleges of Pharmacy.[178] The early pharmacy schools that were the most successful in educating African Americans were Howard University College of Pharmacy and Meharry Pharmaceutical College. From the 1870's until the 1930's, these schools conferred the most pharmacy degrees upon African Americans more than any other programs in the nation. Temple University School of Pharmacy graduated more than 63 African Americans between 1911 and 1926. Xavier University of Louisiana, which opened in 1927, added 195 graduates between 1930 and 1950.[179] (See **Table 3**.) The states' legislature approved the establishment of Texas Southern University School of Pharmacy (1948) and Florida A&M University School of Pharmacy (1951). By the mid-1950s, the number of African American pharmacists from the HBCUs started increasing to the point that today the majority of African Americans with formal pharmacy education graduate from HBCUs.

TABLE 3. Pharmacy Graduates from Xavier College of Pharmacy: 1930–1950

Session	Female Graduates	Male Graduates	Total Graduates
1927–1930	2	6	8
1930–1931	3	3	6
1931–1932	2	9	11
1932–1933	0	2	2
1933–1934	0	6	6
1934–1935	3	5	8
1935–1936	3	9	12
1936–1937	1	1	2
1937–1938	2	3	5
1938–1939	1	5	6
1939–1940	1	2	3
1940–1941	1	6	7
1941–1942	0	3	3
1942–1943	0	3	3
1943–1944	2	4	6
1944–1945	2	1	3
1945–1946	3	2	5
1946–1947	3	6	9
1947–1948	2	7	9
1948–1949	4	22	26
1949–1950	6	49	55
Total	**41 (21%)**	**154 (79%)**	**195**

Sources: Xavier College Bulletins, 1929-1940. Xavier University Bulletin, General Catalogue Number for the Academic Years: 1941-1950. Sisters of the Blessed Sacrament: New Orleans, LA.

2 Meharry Pharmaceutical College

John E. Clark, Trudy Kelly

Meharry Medical College in Nashville, Tennessee is one of the nation's oldest and largest historically black academic health science centers. The school was formed in 1865 by the work of the Methodist Episcopal Church during the Reconstruction period after the Civil War. The church created a mission school for former slaves in a small building known as Andrew Chapel in Nashville. The attendance grew so large during the first year, the school had to be move to a larger building known as the "Gun Factory," which was abandoned property confiscated by the Federal government during the Civil War. The Freedmen Bureau donated the furniture for the school. A Board of Trustees was organized, and a charter was procured from the Tennessee state legislature. In 1865, the school was incorporated as the Central Tennessee College.[180] The Missionary Society of the Methodist Episcopal Church gave the Board of Trustees $11,500 to purchase a site and erect a new building for the college, as the Gun Factory building was a temporary location. A new site was purchased for the school and several buildings erected. In 1872, Dr. George Whipple Hubbard and Dr. John Braden conceived the idea of training African American doctors to take care of their own people. By 1873, Dr. Braden had begun formulating a plan to attach a medical department to the school. In 1876, the Medical Department of Central Tennessee College was started after a $30,000 timely donation was provided for an endowment by the Meharry brothers.[181] It was at this time the Medical Department became the first health science school in the South for training African American physicians and later included dentists, pharmacists, and nurses. The school was named in honor of the Meharry brothers – Samuel Meharry, Alexander Meharry, David Meharry, Jesse Meharry, and Hugh Meharry – for their generous financial support, positive inspiration, and deep interest in uplifting African Americans.[182] (See **Figure 6**.) Aided by the Rev. R.S. Rust, corresponding Secretary of the Freedmen's Aid Society of the Methodist Episcopal Church, the first Medical College building was erected in 1879.[183]The name of the college was changed in 1900 to the Meharry Medical College of Walden University in honor of the Rev. John M. Walden, Bishop of the Methodist Episcopal Church and the principal organizer of the Freedmen's Aid Society. On October 13, 1915, it received a separate charter from the State of Tennessee and was renamed the Meharry Medical College, as it exists today.[184]

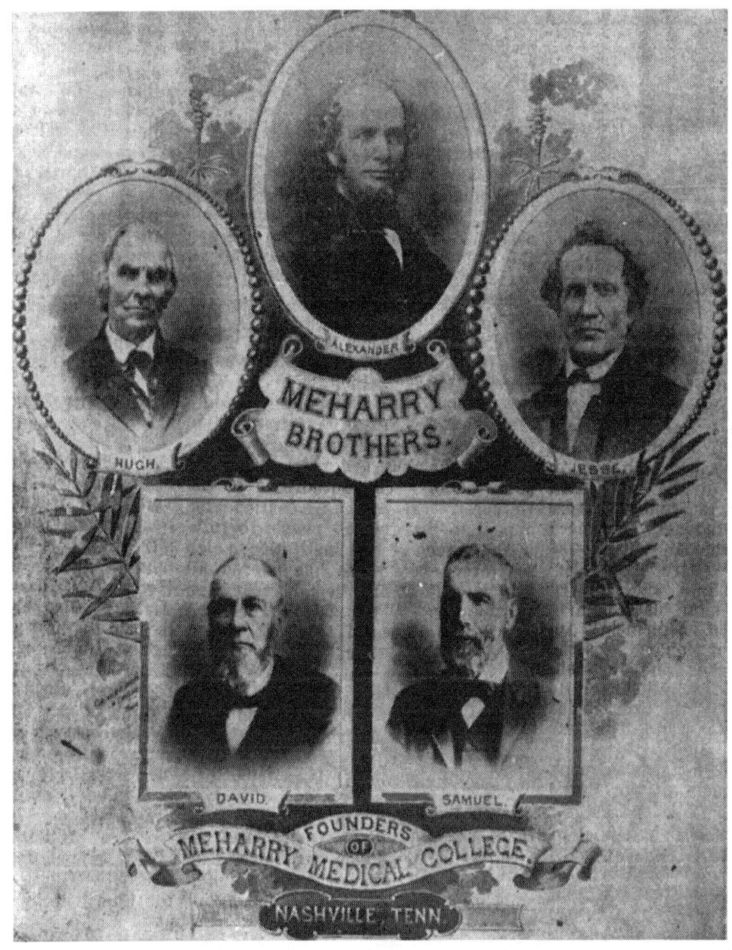

FIGURE 6. The Meharry Brothers.

(Source: *Nashville Globe*, April 25, 1913)

The Meharry Pharmaceutical College was formed as a Department of the Meharry Medical College in 1889. The pharmacy program was first announced in the Spring at the end of the 1889–1890 session, but did not officially enroll students until September 1890.[185] Initially, the program could be completed in two sessions, with each session being 20 weeks long at a tuition cost of $25.00 per session.[186] At the beginning of the 1895–1896 session, the program was extended to 3 sessions and the tuition cost increased to $30.00 per session.[187]

The pharmacy program initially had the same admission requirements as the Medical College,[188] which included: (1) pre-examination in the subjects of English, Arithmetic, Algebra, Physics, and Latin; (2) the candidates had to be of good moral character; and (3) the candidates had to be at least 18 years of age.[189] The school had no gender-based or race-based admission policy. Since its opening, women were admitted using the same criteria as men. (See **Figure 7**.)

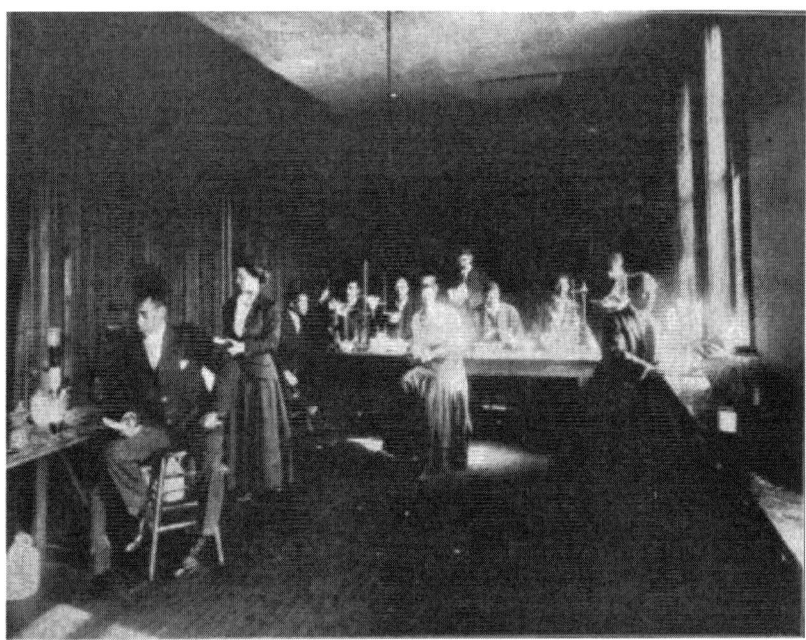

FIGURE 7. African American Women in the Pharmaceutical Laboratory at Meharry Pharmacy College.

(Source: Meharry Medical College, "1910 Meharry Medical College Catalogue," *Meharry Medical College Archives*, accessed January 4, 2016, http://diglib.mmc.edu/omeka/items/show/103.)

To graduate: (1) students had to be twenty-one years of age, be of a good moral character, and have attended all sessions in full at the school; (2) they had to pass an examination with a satisfactory score in each class within the course, including an examination on the outline of Bible history and its doctrine; and (3) they had to have four years of practical experience, inclusive of the sessions in the pharmacy course, in compounding and dispensing drugs and medicines in an established pharmacy.[190] Upon full completion of all requirements, the Graduate of Pharmacy (Ph.G.) degree was conferred.[191] For those completing the pharmacy program, but not meeting the pharmacy practice requirement, a pharmacy certificate (PC) was issued until the practice requirements were met. By 1896, the Ph.G. degree was no longer being offered. Instead, the college began awarding the Pharmaceutical Chemist (Ph.C.) degree for those who successfully completed the requirements for graduation.[192]

The Pharmaceutical College faculty at Meharry was made up of primarily medical doctors (M.D.) from the Medical College. From 1890 to 1900, approximately 80% of the teaching in the Pharmaceutical College was done by faculty with the M.D., Ph.D., and other non-pharmacy degrees. (See **Table 4**.)

TABLE 4. Meharry Pharmaceutical College: Percent of Faculty by Degree: 1890–1935

Session	M.D.	M.D., Ph.C., Ph.G.	Ph.C., Ph.G.	Other (AM, DDS, BS, Ph.D., etc.)
1890–1900	38.3	6.4	12.8	42.6
1901–1909	44	20	16	20
1910–1919	37.3	17.9	43.3	1.5
1920–1934	50.2	5.1	30	14.7

Sources: Meharry Medical College. Meharry Medical College Catalogues, 1890-1935. Nashville, TN: *Meharry Medical College Archives*, accessed March 3, 2016, http://diglib.mmc.edu/omeka/items/browse?collection=3.

On February 1, 1921, Dr. John J. Mullowney was installed as President of Meharry Medical College, succeeding Dr. George W. Hubbard. One of the significant improvements he made shortly after taking charge was the separation of the medical teaching from the teaching of dentistry and pharmacy.[193] Between 1921–1925, the pharmacy curriculum was changed to a two semester system and the length of the curriculum also increased to a three-year program.[194] (See **Table 5** and **Figure 8**.)

TABLE 5. Meharry Pharmaceutical College Courses and Hours: 1928–1929

First Year	**Lectures**	**Laboratory**
Pharmacy	64	464
General Chemistry	32	160
Qualitative Chemistry	32	96
Pharmaceutical Chemistry	30	0
Pharmacognosy	64	0
Physiology	64	0
Hygiene	48	0
Botany	32	112
Total	366	832
Second Year	**Lectures**	**Laboratory**
Materia Medica	96	0
Organic Chemistry	96	240
Operative Pharmacy	32	96
U.S.P. Testing	16	80
Urinalysis	—	—
Therapeutics	32	—
Toxicology	64	—
Pharmaceutical Chemistry	32	176
Pharmacognosy	64	224
Total	432	816
Third Year	**Lectures**	**Laboratory**
Dispensing	64	160
Food and Drug Analysis	64	432
U.S.P. Assaying	64	384
Commercial Pharmacy	48	—

Bacteriology	80	216
Organic Pharmacy	48	0
Total	368	1192
Total Lectures and Laboratory	1166	2840

Source: Meharry Medical College, "1929 Meharry Medical College Catalogue," *Meharry Medical College Archives*, accessed April 8, 2018, http://diglib.mmc.edu/omeka/items/show/118.

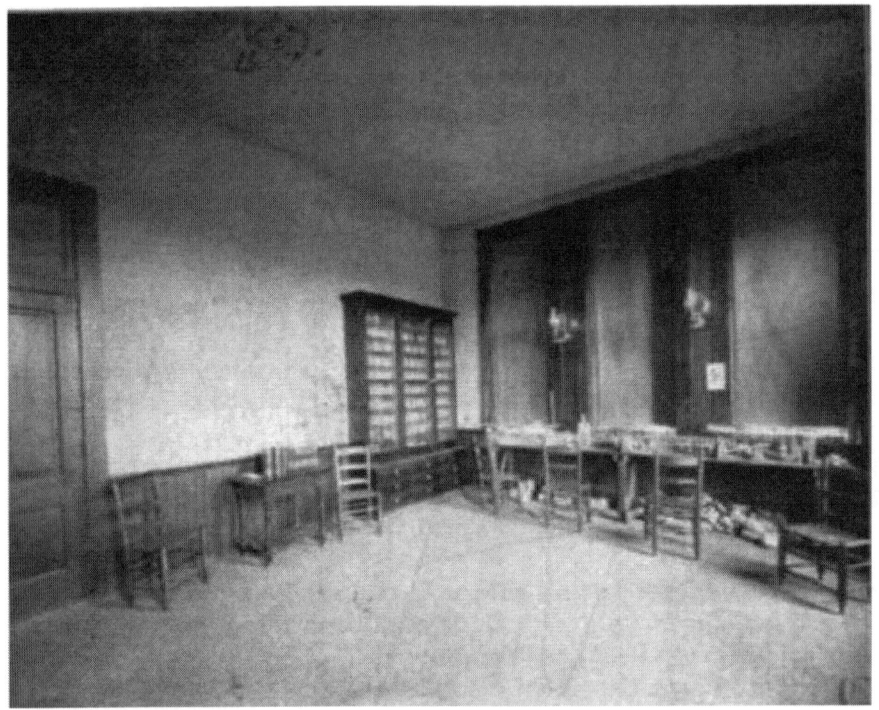

FIGURE 8. Pharmaceutical Recitation Room.

(Source: Meharry Medical College , "1899 Meharry Medical College Catalogue," *Meharry Medical College Archives*, accessed November 18, 2019, http://diglib.mmc.edu/omeka/items/show/92.)

By 1928, the enrollment of pharmacy students had also increased. The Pharmaceutical College was reorganized to create a Division of Pharmacy where much of the teaching was done by pharmacy-trained faculty with Ph.C. and Ph.G. degrees.[195] The Head of the Division of Pharmacy was Wiley C. Baines, Ph.C., a 1921 graduate of the University of Minnesota College of Pharmacy.[196] (See **Figure 9**.). Additional faculty included G. W. Bugg, Jr., Ph.C. and G. C. Lark, Ph.C., B.S. Mr. Baines succeeded Dr. William Sevier, M.D., Ph.G., a Meharry pharmacy alumnus, who had been in charge of the Pharmacy Department for many years and was honorably mention as "one of the most colorful personalities that Meharry has produced."[197] He was well recognized for instilling into students high professional standards and core values of professionalism that encompassed his legacy. (See **Figure 10**.)

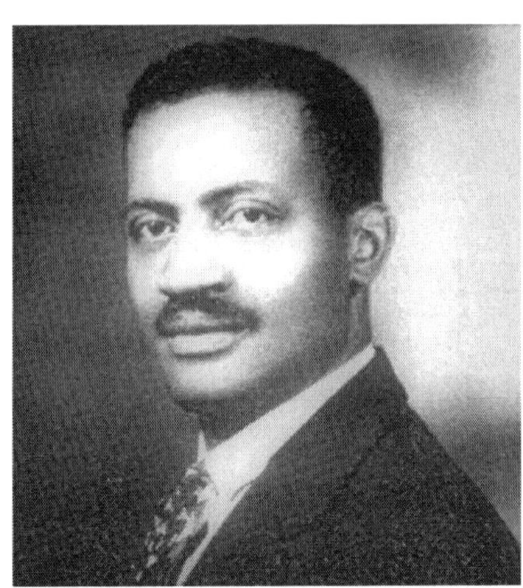

FIGURE 9. Mr. Wiley C. Baines, Head of Pharmacy Department, Meharry Pharmaceutical College.

(Source: Charles Victor Roman, *Meharry Medical College: A History* [Nashville, TN: Sunday School Publishing Board of the National Baptist Convention, Inc., 1934], 157.)

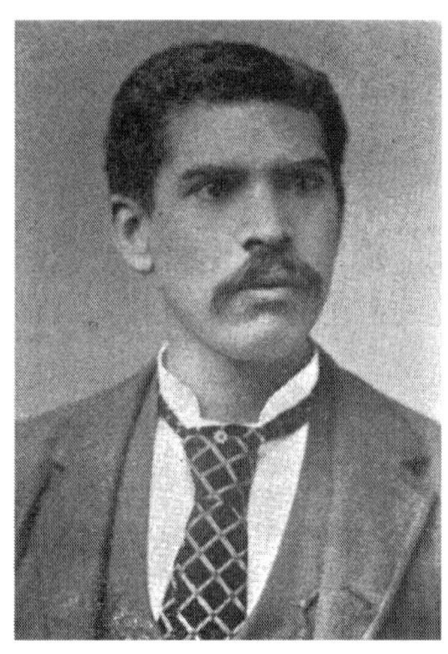

FIGURE 10. Dr. William Sevier, Former Head of the Pharmacy Department, Meharry Pharmaceutical College.

(Source: Charles Victor Roman, *Meharry Medical College: A History* [Nashville, TN: Sunday School Publishing Board of the National Baptist Convention, Inc., 1934], 158.)

The Pharmaceutical College reached its peak in student enrollment and graduates between 1916–1925. (See **Table 6**.) The average number of graduates was approximately 20 students per year. Enrollment started declining after the 1928 session. (See **Figure 11**.). At the beginning of the 1935–1936 session, it was announced that unless 20 students register for the 1936 freshman class, an announcement will be made to all prospective applicants that a satisfactory number has not sought admission to the pharmacy department to warrant a freshman class for the 1936–1937 session. When the enrollment failed to reach 20 students, the pharmacy program ended with the graduation of the 1936 class. No pharmacy classes were offered for the 1936–1937 session, and thereafter.[198]

TABLE 6. Pharmacy Graduates from Meharry Pharmaceutical Department: 1890–1936

Session	Students Enrolled No. (%)	Total Graduates No. (%)
1890–1895	55 (65)	30 (35)
1896–1905	148 (72.2)	54 (27.9)
1906–1915	287 (68.3)	133 (31.7)
1916–1925	539 (73.4)	194 (26.6)
1926–1936	384 (72.6)	146 (27.4)
Total	**1413 (71.7)**	**557 (28.3)**

Sources: Meharry Medical College, "1925 Meharry Medical College Catalogue," *Meharry Medical College Archives*, accessed December 23, 2015, http://diglib.mmc.edu/omeka/items/show/114. Meharry Medical College, "1935 Meharry Medical College Catalogue," *Meharry Medical College Archives*, accessed December 23, 2015, http://diglib.mmc.edu/omeka/items/show/124.

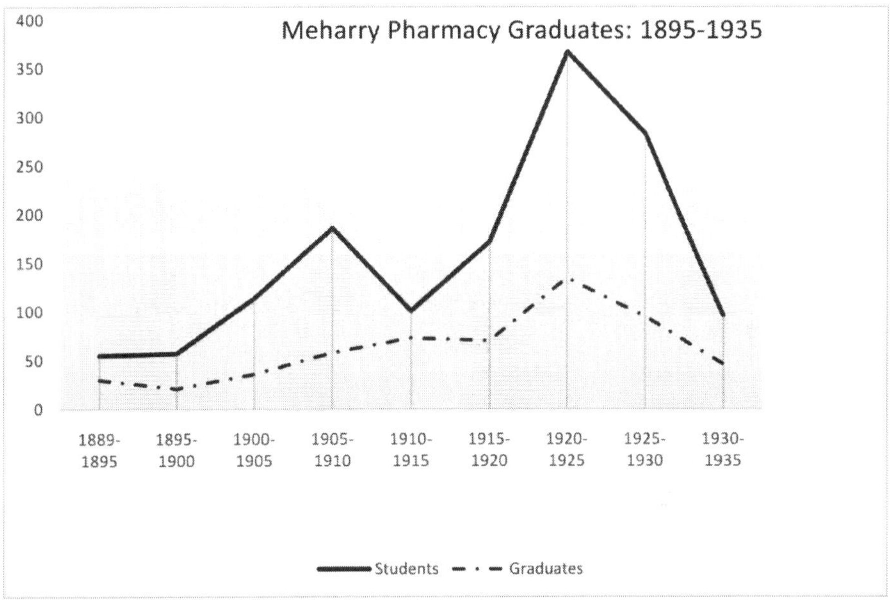

FIGURE 11. African American Pharmacy Graduates from Meharry by Year.

(Sources: Meharry Medical College, "1925 Meharry Medical College Catalogue," *Meharry Medical College Archives*, accessed December 23, 2015, http://diglib.mmc.edu/omeka/items/show/114. Meharry Medical College, "1935 Meharry Medical College Catalogue," *Meharry Medical College Archives*, accessed December 23, 2015, http://diglib.mmc.edu/omeka/items/show/124)

Meharry Pharmaceutical College had the most significant impact on the education of African American pharmacists in the South. Between 1890 and 1936, Meharry graduated more than 550 African American pharmacists, of whom 82 (15%) were women. (See **Table 7**.)

TABLE 7. Pharmacy Graduates from Meharry Pharmaceutical Department by Gender: 1890–1936

Session	Females No. (%)	Males No. (%)
1890–1895	4 (13.3)	26 (86.7)
1896–1905	15 (26.3)	39 (73.7)
1906–1915	21 (15.8)	112 (84.2)
1916–1925	25 (11.8)	169 (88.2)
1926–1936	17 (11.1)	129 (88.9)
Total	**82 (14.7)**	**475 (85.3)**

Sources: Meharry Medical College, "1925 Meharry Medical College Catalogue," *Meharry Medical College Archives*, accessed December 23, 2015, http://diglib.mmc.edu/omeka/items/show/114. Meharry Medical College, "1935 Meharry Medical College Catalogue," *Meharry Medical College Archives*, accessed December 23, 2015, http://diglib.mmc.edu/omeka/items/show/124.

Most of the pharmacy graduates (greater than 66%) remained in the South. (See **Figure 12**.) There, they filled a void that was sorely needed due to the large underserved African American communities in the South, but many went on to be employed and to open drugstores throughout the U.S. for the first time. In a 1934 survey, it was reported that 75% of Meharry pharmacy graduates were gainfully employed; 15% owned and operated their own drugstores; and about 10% were lost to follow-up.[199] A small percentage of the pharmacy graduates also went back to medical school and spent their careers working as physicians. Of the 36 graduates in the first six pharmaceutical classes (1890–1895), 15 subsequently studied medicine and started a medical practice.[200] By the time the school graduated its last class in 1936,[201] it had awarded the largest number of pharmacy degrees to African Americans in the country, including delivering one of the largest number of African American female graduates into the profession of pharmacy. (See **Table 7**.)

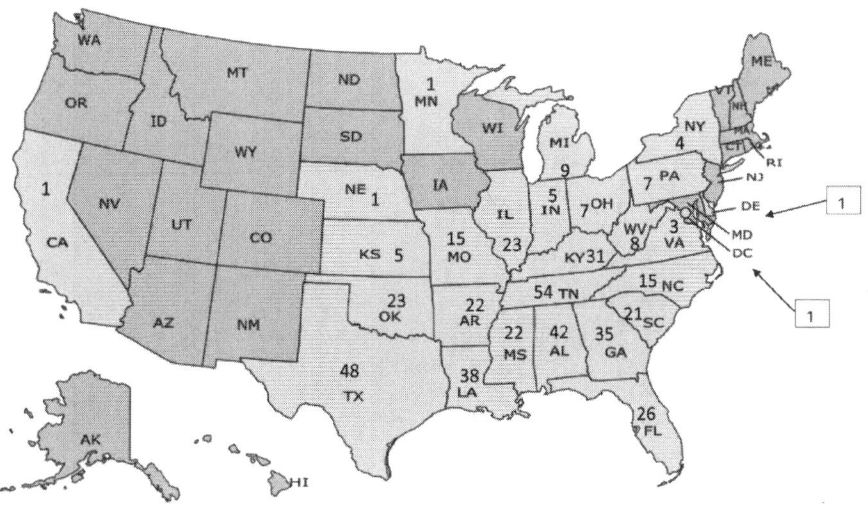

FIGURE 12. Geographical Distribution of Meharry Pharmacy Graduates: 1890–1931.

(Source: Meharry Medical College, "1930 Meharry Medical College Catalogue," *Meharry Medical College Archives*, accessed December 28, 2015, http://diglib.mmc.edu/omeka/items/show/119.)

TABLE 8. Graduates of the Meharry Pharmaceutical College, 1890–1936

CLASS	NAME	
1890	Hobbs, John T.	
1891	Allen, Robert W.	
	Beverly, James M.	
	Randals, Edward S.	
1892	Armistead, Henry W.	
	Sevier, William	
	Tyler, Robert	
1893	Crawford, J. P.	Smith, F.G.
	Crutchfield, G. K	Simms, W.H.
	Coffin, F.B.	Williams, R. C.
1894	Coleman (Winston), Ella E.	Samuel, A. L.

CLASS	NAME	
1894	Caffey, Frank C.	Simington, Alfred D.
	Jennings, Joseph J.	Smith, Charles H.
	Lloyd, Matilda	Wendell, Thomas T.
	Miller (Redfield), Margaret A.	Washington, George E.
	Rowland, W.	Winston, Samuel J
1895	Bailey, W.H.	Kigh, Isaiah
	Joyce, Nannie B.	Watkins, I.S.
	Kelley C.A.	
1896	Easter, B. F.	Lewis, L. W.
	Gowdey, C. E.	McBroom, F. G.
	Johnson D. L.	Morrow (Johnson), Pauline S.
1897	Davis, John C.	Moore (Goin), Bellina A.
	Gaines, J.W.	Parker, A. A.
1898	Brown, Ernest W.	
	Jerry, Z. J.	
	Smith, D. McCoy	
1899	Allen, Griffin A	Lancaster, W. Harvey
	Dean, Ulysses S.	Martin (Dukes), Willie F. L.
	Dejoie, Aristide R.	Taylor, Daniel B.
1900	Jackson, Flossie E.	
1901	Derrick, Thomas H.	Plair, S. M.
	Dumas, H. J.	Sunday, P. M.
	Faulkner, E. L.	Thomas (Hill), Ida B.
	Halston, W. A.	
1902	Barrett, O. B. L.	Foster, James.
	Brown, L. W.	Smith, Minnie L.
	Byrd, D. W.	Breedlove (Taylor), Mabelle A.
1903	Jones, A. T	Moore, T. P.
	Logan, A. L	Ridley (Blackwell), Mattie L.
	McCoy (Johnson), E. Estelle	Turner, E. M.
1904	Bright, J. W.	Thompson, W. S.
	Craig, G. P.	Wilson, A. A.

CLASS	NAME	
1904	Hughes, Annie L.	Winston, James W.
	Mack (Singleton), Sarah E.	
1905	Haynes, William	Rivers, Mayme B.
	Howard, Maggie E.	Thomas, Zenia M.
	Kellix, Lizzie B.	White, H. C.
	LaBranche, E. J.	White, James
1906	Cardwell, E, D.	McKay, F. H.
	Heffron, F. S.	Thompson (Smith), Pearl L.
	Hampton, Zenobia L.	Wilhite, C. A.
	Marble, Harriet	Wilson, Wm. K.
	Miles, Neil	
1907	Durroh, W. T.	Stone, Emma L.
	McIntosh, Erskin	Wallace, W. A.
	Pickens, John L.	Williamson, E. T.
	Ruddock, C. B.	Williams, J. B.
1908	Alford, M. C.	Love, L. F.
	Anderson, M. S.	Sharp, C. L.
	Bowden, J. M.	Watson, Lillie C. G.
1909	Blount, Lulu S.	Jenkins, Natalie G.
	Dier, C. A.	Kyles, J. G.
	English, J. S.	Nicholson, A. C.
	Franklin, G. W.	Peterson, G. D.
	Gregory, J. A.	Riley, Jennie D.
	Hinson, A. L	Tatum, Katie C. C.
	Harris, E. D.	Thompson, P. S.
	Hightower, J. R.	Thompson, E. T.
	Johnson, R. G.	Walker, Day Beulah L.
1910	Bryant, Hattie Belle	Martin, J.B.
	Foster, Wm. H.	Maclin, Gustava D.
	Foulkes, G. C	Miller, Luther L.
	Grant, M.A.	Mitchell, L. A.
	Gordon, Isaac	O'Bryant, W. E.
	Granberry, D. B.	Peters, Robt. L.
	Granberry, Ruby C.	Williams, Thomas, Jr.
	Jones, Andrew M., M.D	Williams, Willie
	Goodloe, Annie Mae	

CLASS	NAME	
1911	Allison, W. H.	McClain, Jonathan
	Bullock, Gertrude	Perdue, Omar
	Cogbill, H. P.	Pitts, W. A.
	Clarke, H. A.	Reynolds, Elizabeth C.
	Carter, T. C.	Rice, C. C.
	Dockett, Alfred	Stewart, W. J.
	Douglas, H. G.	Taylor, J. A.
	Kellar, W. E.	Turner, S. E.
	Lee, Scottie P.	Wilson, C. A.
	Miller, Ewing	Warren, R. G.
1912	Commons, J. W.	King, M. M. C.
	Dantzler, L. M.	Maxwell, A. E.
	Garner, S. C.	Payne, A. B.
	Gaines, L. B.	Smith, T. M.
	Ivey, W. S.	Stilson, E. L.
	Johnson, T. W., Jr.	Sawyer, J. H.
	Jones, P. D., Jr.	Thompson, W. E.
	Jenkins, M. F.	Wilson, L. S.
	Kennedy, J. A.	
1913	Adams, David A.	Ledbetter, Benji. F.
	Coleman, Senator R.	Phillips, Edward, A.
	Durham, Edwin H.	Patterson, Wm A.
	Dye, M. E.	Reid, Sandy H.
	Ferguson, Abraham L.	Richie, Wm. F.
	Ford, Florence T.	Taylor, Norton
	Goodwin, Aaron W.	Thomas, Charles A.
	Houston, Andrew J.	Thomas, James W.
	Johnson, Samuel O.	Thompson, Earlin
	Lee, Alexander	Wright, John D.
1914	Barbary (Berry), Lelia Pearl	McCollum, N.
	Cravens, E. H.	Randolph, W. W.
	Floyd, C. C.	Shockley, A. C.
	Longdon, R. H.	Taylor, T. M.
1915	Berry, Clifton	Jones, Robbie D. A.
	Baker, D. G	Roberts, W. A.
	Chandler, Wm. E.	Smith, P. N.
	Counts, D.	Sawyer, Gussie L.
	DeLashwa, T. L.	Wright, Reanna Mae

CLASS	NAME	
1916	Artist, Robinson	Kyles, Richie Belle
	Bright, Andrew J.	Morris, Agnes Penelope Whiteman
	Clapp, Claud D.	McGee, Osia
	Clark, Nathaniel	Powell, Jake C.
	Drew, Roy E.	Rawls, James W.
	Goodson, Jeff D., Jr.	Thomasas, Fortune T.
	Harris, Lawrence C.	Turner, Isaiah S.
	Hill, J.S.	Williams, Thomas R.
	Hockett, W. S.	
1917	Bayler, E. M.	McSayles, H. R.
	Boulware, H. T.	Meadors, W. M.
	Clark (Gilmer), Johnnie Etta	Montgomery, W. M.
	Cabell, Delmo B.	Ragan, U. S.
	Cummings, Pearl Esther	Ragland, R. M.
	Dickens, E. L.	Sylvester, H. L.
	Dinkins, Daisy Dorine	Tandy, J. F.
	Donaseur, P. E.	Tycer, B. L.
	Durroh, W. F.	Van Buren, J. L.
	Freeman, W. C.	Vaughn, W. L.
	Hoff, A. H.	Williams, Annie Ruth
	Holliday, J. A.	Williamson, S. T., Jr.
	Lytle, W. H.	
1918	Cook, D. B.	Reid, J. W.
	Coffee, E. B.	Scott, W. S.
	Irving, T. A.	Simpkins, W. V.
	Johnson, Phillip B.	
1919	Egester, J. W. Jr.	Lewis, O. C.
	Gathings, John	Scott, D. E.
	Keene, R. D.	
1920	Beverly, Inez E.	Smith, Horance W.
	Brown, H. N.	Stanton, R. B.
	Lockley, C. J.	Torrence, Naomi H.
	Marshall, H. E.	Williams, F. B.
	Reaed, J. Edwin	Williams, L. S.
	Robinson, Alexander	Wimberly, R. E.
	Sheley, J. K.	

CLASS	NAME	
1921	Benfield, C. L.	Lockridge, Marshall
	Brooks, George S.	Meadors, George S.
	Bryant, Oreba M.	Moore, Maceo
	Carter, Edward A. P.	Pillow (Akin), Ida
	Crothwait, Holcombe S.	Raines (Clay), Lela
	Douglas, Simon R.	Richardson, Edward
	Goff, Granville W.	Schroder, E. L.
	Hale, Eugene W.	Spence, William R.
	Harris, Froncell C.	William, Lee Roy E.
	Hendricks, T. C.	
1922	Alston, Moses J.	Mitchell (Partee), Retha
	Andrews, Samuel, A., Jr.	Nall, James B.
	Blaine, Charles B.	Payne, Rodger D.
	Blakemore, Georgia A.	Partee, Arthur A.
	Bowman, Jameson C.	Ramsey, Claude G.
	Butler, Thomas J.	Reed, Lincoln A.
	Byers, Virgil B.	Richie, Wallace A.
	Buckner, Esquire	Ruff, James R.
	Coleman, John B.	Sartor, Lillian
	Gaillard, George O.	Sisson, Larnie H.
	Gordon (Andrews), Sallie I.	Shines (Wood), Wilhelmina E.
	Harden, Early Lee	Thornton, Handsome
	Harper, Mildred G.	Tillman, Ernest A.
	Harris, Thomas M.	Varnadoe, Drusilla A.
	Hoyle, Lewis M.	Washington, A. Nathaniel
	Kiser, Thomas P.	Williams, Herbert R.
	Lindsay, Alvin	Williams, Rufus J.
	Maney, A. Z.	Williams, William O.
	McIntyre, M. B.	Wood, Clarence N.
1923	Baylor, Chester Thomas..	Livingston, William McKinley
	Benjamin, Louis	McDonald, Walter Isaac
	Bundy, Van Gilbert	Nelson, Hosea Caesar
	Campbell, Thomas Nelson	Pierce, Raymond Olee
	Carter, Elmer Milton	Rayford, Samuel Simeon
	Cook, William Henry, Jr.	Richardson, Levan Whittier
	Dunnings, Otis M.	Roberts, Clarence LaFayette
	Eigner, Chester Arthur	Sales, Robert Turner
	Evans, Noble	Simpson, William Emmanuel
	Jackson, Dorothy Lois	Wallace, Clarence E.
	Jenkins, Joseph Wiley	Wallace, Lee Lucky

CLASS	NAME	
1923	Jones, Isom W.	Williams, Bertha L.
	Jordon, Adolph Eugene	Young, James Willie
	King, Leronious J.	Young, Noble Ernest
	Lewis, George P.	
1924	Baker, Edwin	Greenwood, Augustus Marion
	Blanchet, Cleolus Leonidas	Harris, Mary Blayne
	Boalware, Theodore Roosevelt	Lyons, Mack
	Bowles, Preston Sewell	Pickett, Elmer Reid
	Bowman, Theodore Roosevelt	Russell, Carrie Nell
	Brown, Harrison B.	Smith, Edward, Hammond
	Collins, James Allen	Strozier, Frank Rogers
	Dickerson, Edward Ernest	White, Sol
	Ervin, Lealand Merrill	Williston, Frank Douglas
	Firmin, Albert Leonard	Wright, Antonio Maceo
	Fredd, Ira Milton	
1925	Alston, Alford Armstrong	Pendergrass, Carrie Belle
	Anderson, Eddie Douglas	Philpott, Frederick
	Bloom, Herbert Lawrence	Printers, Jesse Boyd
	Covington, Lois Vivian	Prewitt, Arthur Carl
	Cox, Oscar Lee	Sampson, Clarence R.
	Gary, Clement Mantell	Scott, Charles E.
	Hausman, Oliver Joseph	Taylor, LaVaunt
	Hillard, Fred	Thomas, James Edward
	Hunt, Thomas	Thompkins, Frederick J.
	Le Mon, Harrison H.	Wells, Edward G.
	McKnight, Amos Charles	Young, Ulysses S.
1926	Allen, James Lucius	Langford, Edgar A.
	Cabell, Roger W.	Logan, John A.
	Carlisle, Wilburn T.	McCain (Young), Georgia M.
	Eaverly, Wallace	Moore Dewey
	Force, James Hill	Patton, Davye Lee
	Foster, C. Myrtle	Preear, Richard P.
	Golden, Alexander H.	Seawell (Crawford), R. Lulu
	Harden, Julius C. H.	Thornton, Clarence C.
	Jackson, Frank A.	Trimble, Cecil C.
	Jones, Cunighan S.	Wilkins, Edwyn Jos.
	Jones, Herbert W.	Williams, Francis W.
	Jones, Isaac I.	Witherspoon, Edward A.
	Jones, James W.	Woods, Wm. P. G.

CLASS	NAME	
1926	Lange, Arthur H.	
1927	Barnett, David W.	Mason, Clarence Benjamin
	Buford, Bert	Morrison, McLean Joseph
	Gibbs, Wilmote D.	Neal, Xenophon L.
	Harris, Tolliver	Smith, Viola M.
	Hudson, James B.	Williams, Carl Chatman
	Jones, Dorothy Bennett	Windham (Buford), Corinne
	McDonald, Jerome Eldridge	Young, Robert Theodore
	Martin, Titus J.	
1928	Austin, Lillian D.	Lewis (Blanchett), Mollie V.
	Bennett, Ridgely C.	Marshall, Robert S.
	Browning, W. D.	Martin, Theodore G.
	Bryant, Moses	Mills, Otis J.
	Collins Albert T.	Slack, John L.
	Donnegan, W. G.	Taylor, Harvey R.
	Freeman, E. Lamar	Trezevant, L. E.
	French, Shelton	Vick, Samuel H., Jr.
	Hilliburton, G. W.	Wiggins, Albert
	Hunter, William C.	Wynn, Thomas C.
	Jones, Henrietta Clara	Young, Horace M.
	Knox, Thomas J.	
1929	Bugg, George W., Jr.	Perkins, Bernard
	Davis, Wadsworth A.	Pinkney, John H., Jr.
	French, Wendell M.	Purvis, L. T.
	Gallimore, Lonnie	Richardson, Toby
	Jackson, Osceola	Ross, A. W.
	Jacobs, James W.	Shepard, Thurston J.
	Morrell, E. M.	Washington, James S.
	Patterson, Ernest E.	Wesley, Mavis P.
1930	Aycock, Joe Olney	Perry, William R.
	Clardy, Edgar	Price, Eugene L., Jr.
	Cotton, Rutlin H.	Rhodes, Lucie Lee
	Crawley, Thomas O.	Riddick, Hortense Iona
	Fisher, Robert H.	Smart, Lillian Burton
	Kendall, Chauncey	Smith, Sidney Earl
	Moore, Columbus Vernon	Winters, Henry H.
1931	Beverly, Carter C.	Hill, Harold E.

CLASS	NAME	
1931	Black Jerome W.	LeGall, Fitzherbert H.
	Brown, Miss. S. DeWitt	Mosby, W. Houston
	Clarke, Ernest J.	McFall, John A., Jr.
	Duncan, Goodwin W.	Walker, Jerome
	Fitzgerald, Herman	Weems, Joseph J.
1932	Baldwin, Samuel H.	Neal, Richard Maurice
	Benson, Mrs. Georgia W.	Parham, Glover P.
	Grant, Randolph O.	Ray, Alvin K.
	Gudger, Alfred	Reid, C. A.
	Haddox, Morris B.	Wallace, W. Boyd
	Jones, Thomas A.	Woodson, S. W.
	Lindsay, Percy A.	
1933	Brown, Jackson H.	Harris, E. D.
	Christopher, Theo M.	Hendricks, Louis
	Fielder, A. L.	James, Lewis
	Hall, Mack	Stewart, James
1934	Boyd, Evalyn R.	
	Reed, M.C.	
1935	Caldwell, Edgar L.	Murray, James A.
	Fowler, Allen G.	Poole, George R.
	Goodloe, T. A.	Settle, Antonio Juan
	Hawthorne, Jonathan	Thomas, Canzy G.
	McNeil, William H.	Webb, Clarence
	Moss, Arthur A.	
1936	Harrington, Roosevelt	
	Johnson, Charles A.	
	Taylor, Daniel E., Jr.	
	Walker, Charles W.	

Source: Meharry Medical College, "1928 Meharry Medical College Catalogue," *Meharry Medical College Archives*, accessed November 22, 2019, http://diglib.mmc.edu/omeka/items/show/117; Meharry Medical College, "1936 Meharry Medical College Catalogue," *Meharry Medical College Archives*, accessed November 22, 2019, http://diglib.mmc.edu/omeka/items/show/125.

Among the notable Meharry pharmacy graduates was *John B. Martin* (1910), aka J.B. Martin,[202] who moved to Memphis after graduation and opened his own drugstore. His business was so successful that it was expanded into a chain of drugstores throughout the South. He owned the popular South Memphis Drug Stores. (See **Figure 13.**) He was also, perhaps, the first African American pharmacist to own two professional baseball teams.[203] J. B. Martin, along with his brothers, William Martin (physician), A.T. Martin, and B.B. Martin (dentist), owned the Memphis Red Sox (1923–1950) and the stadium where the team played. (See **Figure 14**.) Prior to the brothers acquiring the team, the stadium was named Lewis Park, after the architect Robert Lewis, who built the first baseball stadium for blacks in the U.S. It was located on the corner of Crump Boulevard and South Lauderdale Street in Memphis. After the Martins acquired the team, they renovated and changed the name of the stadium to Martin Stadium and used it for not only baseball, but for football games, track and field, and other organized events.[204] This was a major business accomplishment by the Martins and even more so for black entrepreneurs at the time. Most professional teams in the Negro leagues played their games in the white-owned baseball stadiums. In Martin Stadium, the Martins had complete control over the revenue from the baseball team, from the stadium concessions, and from a nearby hotel that they owned. With segregation still a part of daily life, it was also one of the few public places in America that offered a comforting environment where the African American community could attend professional sporting events without the restriction experienced at white-owned stadiums.[205] (See **Figure 15**.) J.B. Martin later moved to Chicago where he served as the President of the Negro American Baseball League and acquired ownership of his second professional baseball team, the Chicago American Giants (1937–1950).[206] After a few years, he sold the team to Abe Saperstein, owner of the Harlem Globetrotters basketball team, and began to pursue a political career. In 1946, he was elected as the first African American member of the Board of Trustees of the Chicago Metropolitan Sanitary District.[307]

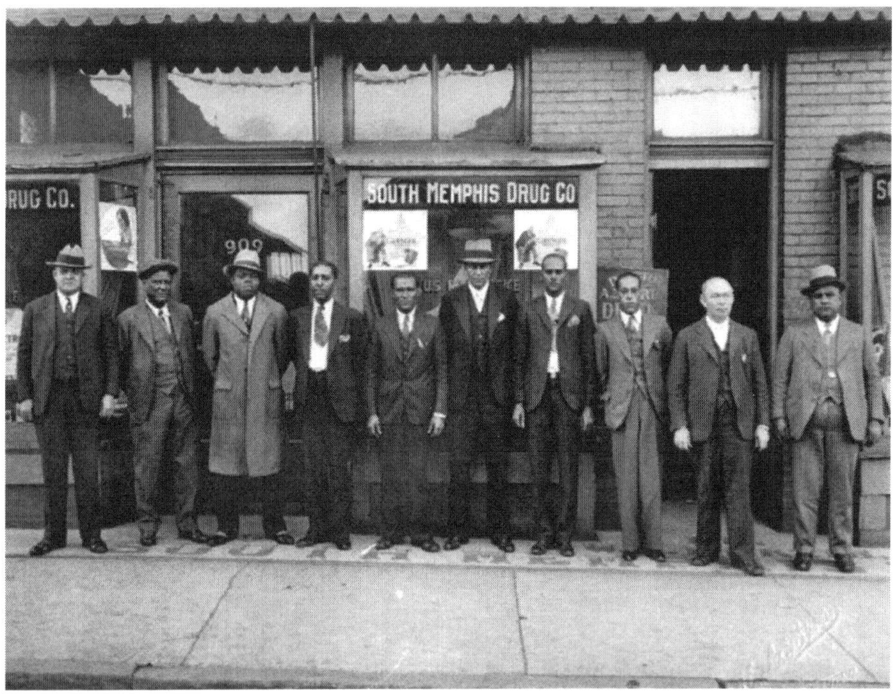

FIGURE 13. J. B. Martin (far left) standing in front of the South Memphis Drug Store, circa 1930s.

(Source: *Historic Drug Stores.....and the Memphis Drug Supply House.* Accessed from: http://historic-memphis.com/memphis-historic/drug-stores/drug-stores.html. March 25, 2016.)

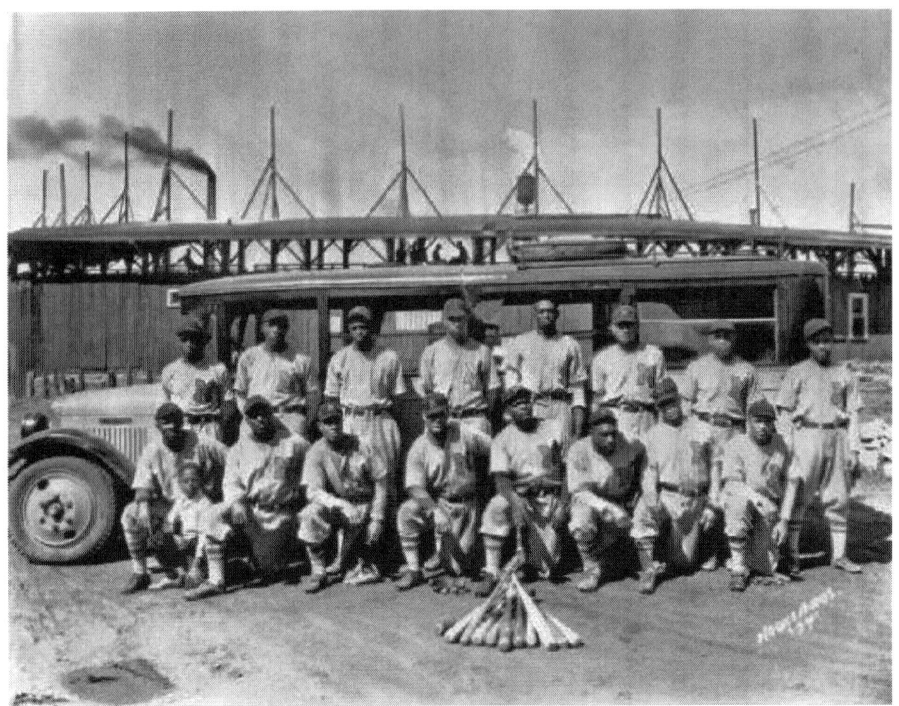

FIGURE 14. Memphis Red Sox baseball team in front of Martin Stadium, circa 1934.

(Source: Jenkins, Ernest Lovelle. *Images of America: African Americans in Memphis,* [Charleston, SC: Arcadia Publishing, 2009], 40.)

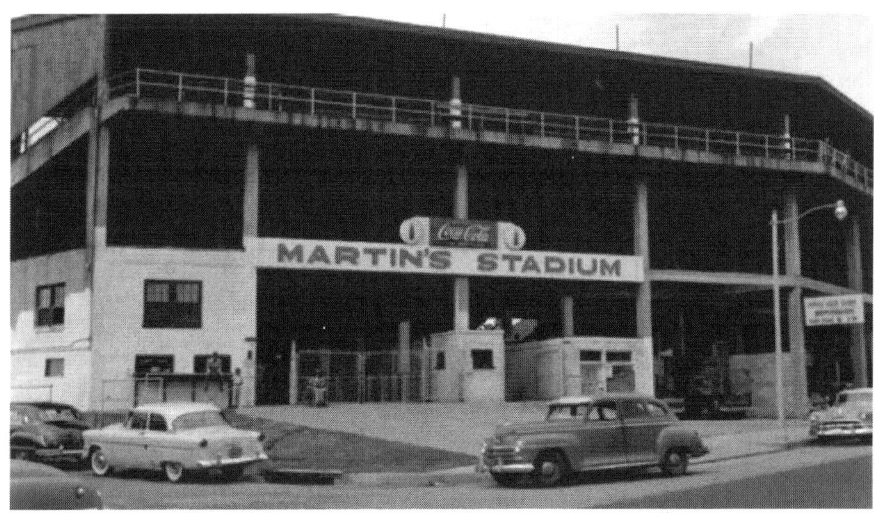

FIGURE 15. Martin Stadium, Home of the Memphis Red Sox.

(Source: *Ernest Wither Collection Museum & Gallery*, 1954; *Coca-Cola Journey*, February 23, 2016, https://www.coca-colacompany.com/stories/photographer-ernest-withers-had-an-eye-on-history--coca-cola)

Other Meharry pharmacy notables include *Ella E. Coleman, Margaret A. Miller, and Matilda Lloyd* who were the first known African American females to be awarded pharmacy degrees in the U.S. They received the Graduate in Pharmacy (Ph.G.) degree in 1894 and it was also the first time that three African American women graduated in the same class in a pharmacy program in the U.S.[208] After graduation, Matilda Lloyd was employed as a member of the faculty at Central Tennessee College in 1898[209] and later joined the executive staff at the Meharry Pharmaceutical College as Assistant Registrar, where she remained for more than 40 years.[210] (See **Figure 16**.) It is unclear whether Ella E. Coleman and Margaret A. Miller were able to get their career started as pharmacists or pursued work in other occupational areas.

Other outstanding female pharmacy graduates were: *Pauline S. Marrow* (1896), the first African American female pharmacist in Victoria, Texas;[211] *Harriet B. Marble* (Ph.C. 1906) was the first African American female pharmacist to open a drugstore in Lexington, Kentucky[212] and one of the first to be a registered pharmacist in four states.[213] (See **Figure 17**.) *Mollie Lewis-Moon* (Ph.C. 1928) was internationally recognized for her involvement in and the founding of the National Urban League Guild;[214] (see **Figure 18**) and *Lillian D. Robinson* (Ph.C. 1928), internationally recognized cosmetologist, beauty consultant, and hair stylist.[214]

Meharry Pharmaceutical College was a member of the American Conference of Pharmaceutical Faculties (ACPF),[215] which indicates that the level of pharmaceutical education provided was of the highest standard at the time. Shortly before the Pharmaceutical College closed in 1936, the administration had approved the changing of the curriculum from a three-year to a four-year degree program, thus continuing to raise the educational standards.

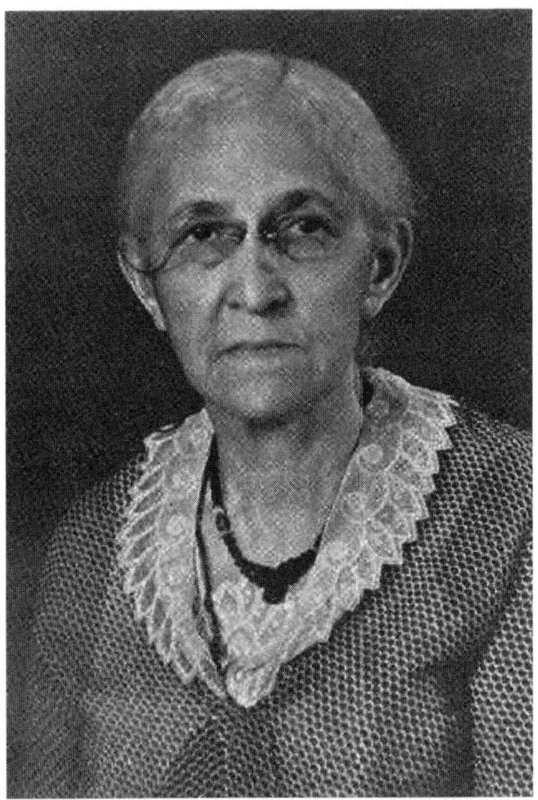

FIGURE 16. Matilda Lloyd, Emeritus Assistant Registrar.

(Source: Charles Victor Roman, *Meharry Medical College: A History* [Nashville, TN: Sunday School Publishing Board of the National Baptist Convention, Inc., 1934], 14.)

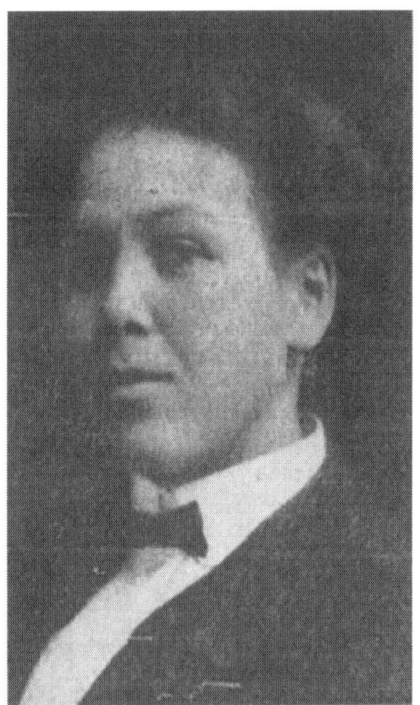

FIGURE 17. Harriet Marble.
(Source: *Nashville Globe*, August 22, 1913.)

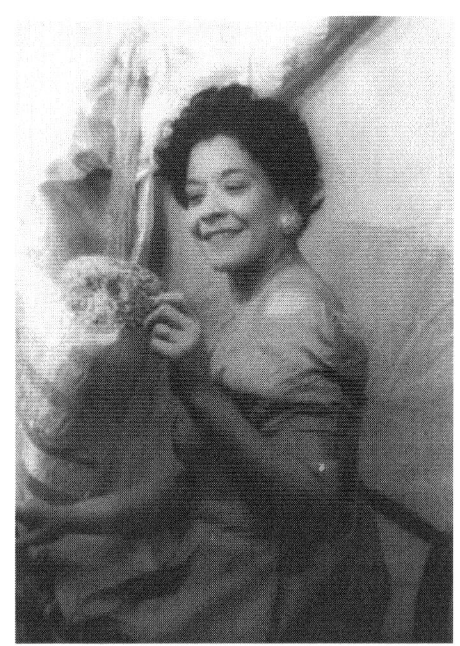

FIGURE 18. Mollie Moon, President, National Urban League Guild, 1956.
(Source: Carl Van Vechten, Photographer, *Wikipedia*.)

3 Shaw University Leonard School of Pharmacy

John E. Clark, Angela M. Hill

Shaw University considered the "crown jewel" of the American Baptist Home Mission Society, was initially known as the Raleigh Baptist Institute. Its inception coincided with the end of the Civil War in 1865 in the city of Raleigh, North Carolina, which had become a congregating point for large numbers of African Americans fleeing the bondage of slavery and the Confederate armies. The school was the brainchild of Mr. Henry Martin Tupper, founder and President of Shaw University and a former chaplain in the Union Army. It was named in honor of Elijah Shaw of Wales, Massachusetts for his generous financial gifts to the institution.

Mr. Tupper was an ordained minister who had much experience with African Americans during the Civil War and a significant understanding of their plight. Since his desire was to create a school for African Americans grounded in Christian education with a spiritual, moral, and intellectual component, much of the classroom education was in theology, although he had long desired to create a school for training African American physicians. By 1880, the need for training in fields other than theology and the timely generous donations by his brother-in-law, led to the creation of a medical department, which was followed by departments of law and pharmacy.

In 1881, the Leonard School of Medicine and Pharmacy at Shaw University were established and approved by the North Carolina legislature.[217]The site for the medical and pharmacy school buildings, as well as a hospital, dispensary, and dormitories for male and female students were contributed by the North Carolina state legislature. Mr. Tupper had to solicit for funds before the building construction could start. He was a very skillful and motivated fundraiser. He campaigned mostly in the North, where he grew up. There he prevailed upon enough people to provide funds and pledges to construct the buildings needed for the schools. He also raised enough to establish endowments for the university. One of several people he honored was his brother-in-law, Judson Wade Leonard, who had given $5,000 toward the establishment of the medical school. He named the School of Medicine and School of Pharmacy in his honor.[218] He also named the Medical School building, the Medical School hospital, and the Dispensary in his name for his additional financial contributions to the development of the programs at the institution. (See **Figure 19**.)

The pharmacy program started at Shaw in 1890 as a three-year course with each session lasting 32 weeks. (See **Table 9**.) The admission requirements were like that of the medical school, but somewhat less clear than other similar pharmacy schools. Students applying for admission:

1. Must have basic knowledge of English and the sciences, as well as, pass a pre-examination in the basic topics. A proficiency in Latin was also required. Students lacking this knowledge were recommended to take courses in the topic before applying.[219]
2. Must be of good moral character; and
3. Be at least 18 years of age (required for medical school, but not mentioned in the pharmacy admission requirements).[220]

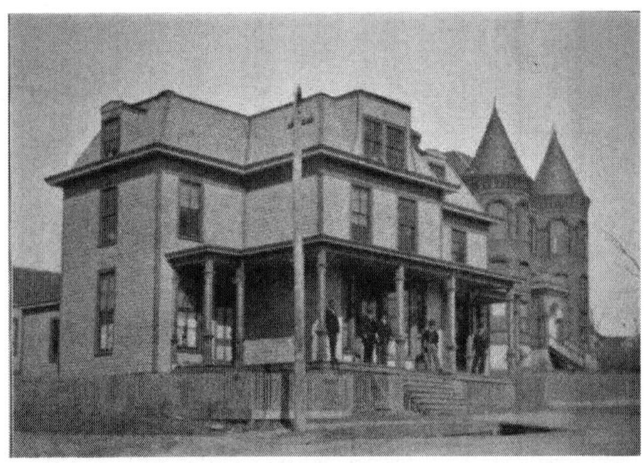

FIGURE 19. Leonard Pharmacy School Building.

(Source: *Ninth Annual Catalog of the Officers and Students of Leonard School of Pharmacy,* Shaw University, 1899.)

TABLE 9. Leonard School of Pharmacy Course Descriptions: 1911–1912

Junior Course

This course embraces a knowledge of the theory of Pharmacy, the sciences involved in the intelligent study and practice of the art, the laws governing the practice of Pharmacy, the Pharmacopoeia of the United States, Pharmacopoeia, Chemical, and Scientific nomenclature, Latin and English Technical Terminology, official and unofficial drugs and preparations, the several systems of weights and measures, embracing also metric system, specific gravity, specific volume, preparation and preservation of drugs; uses and effects of heat, fusion, calcination, sublimation, etc.; solutions of solids, liquids and gases; generation of gases, diffusion, dialysis, extraction, percolation, expression, filtration, other means of separation and purification, evaporation, distillation, crystallization, precipitation, washing, etc. Extemporaneous or Dispensary Pharmacy will be practically illustrated by work done by the students themselves, and for this purpose instruction will be given in preparing official powders, mixtures, emulsions, decoctions, infusions, saturations, etc.

Middle Course

The course of the Middle class will be an advance course to the Junior class, and will comprise the preparation of extracts, fluid extracts, abstracts, pills, spirits, oleates, sealed preparation of iron, troches, ointments, cereates, plasters, suppositories, etc. Instruction in practical training in dispensing will be an important feature in the Middle class, following as closely as possible the outline work commenced in the Junior course. The prescription counter, its management and furnishing, the processes, apparatus, and utensils employed in extemporaneous pharmacy, will be fully discussed and their uses illustrated; also, incompatibility, with special reference to dispensing.

Senior Course

The Senior course will commence with a review of the second year's course, after which the pharmacopoeia preparation will be carefully considered, much time being devoted to the compounding of physicians' prescriptions and extemporaneous pharmacy generally, the assaying of drugs, as opium, cinchona, nux vomica, etc.; practice in the use of specific gravity apparatus, thermometers, alcoholometers, etc.; extraction and preparation of alkaloids and other proximate principles from drugs.

Materia Medica

Detailed study of the substances used medicinally will be accompanied with authentic specimens, that students may become familiar with the appearance of the articles as they are met with in commerce. Notice will be taken of the habitat, commercial history, and official preparation into which the drug enters; also its therapeutic properties, etc. Special attention will be paid to the drilling of students in posology.

Pharmaceutical Laboratory

With the Pharmaceutical Laboratory is combined the Leonard Free Dispensary. Here the student has an excellent opportunity to learn the details of manipulation that make the thorough and practical pharmacist. These are the proper handling and care of apparatus, weighing, the processes of filtration, percolation, etc., the compounding and dispensing of prescriptions, wrapping packages, marking goods, checking invoices, and all the accompanying work with which the druggist must be familiar. Special attention is paid to quickness and accuracy in the making of extemporaneous preparations, such as pills, powders, plasters, and suppositories that are prepared at the prescription counter.

Source: *Twenty-Second Annual Catalog of the Officers and Teachers of the Leonard School of Pharmacy, The Pharmaceutical Department of Shaw University*, (Raleigh, NC: Shaw University, 1912), 45.

The admission policy of the university was open to all, regardless of race and gender.

One of the advantages the Leonard School of Pharmacy claimed to have was the opportunity for students attending their school to acquire pharmacy practice experience on the campus[221] versus trying to acquire the practice experience outside of the school where there may have been significant challenges because of their race.[222] This was made possible because Leonard School of Pharmacy had a pharmaceutical laboratory attached to the Leonard Free Dispensary as part of its classes.[223] In addition to the regular pharmacy courses, the students were given opportunities to gain practical experiences necessary for the preparation of physician's prescriptions from the Leonard Free Dispensary, while they were in school and under the supervision of qualified faculty. (See **Figure 20**.) What is unclear is whether the practice hours were required for graduation.

Two faculty members taught all of the classes until about 1907–1908, when it was increased to three as the student enrollment increased.[224] Most of the faculty who taught in the Leonard School of Pharmacy had pharmacy training and education (i.e., Ph.D., Ph.C. or Ph.G. degrees). (See **Table 10**.) They were also all white men who spent most of their lives in the South or who lived in the northern states of the U.S. and moved to the South. All were at risk for harm by teaching in a school for African Americans. The Ku Klux Klan had threatened Mr. Tupper and his family and expressed bitterness early on to the creation of such a school in the South. Therefore, all who were involved, including teachers and donors, were at risk and mindful of the danger.[225]

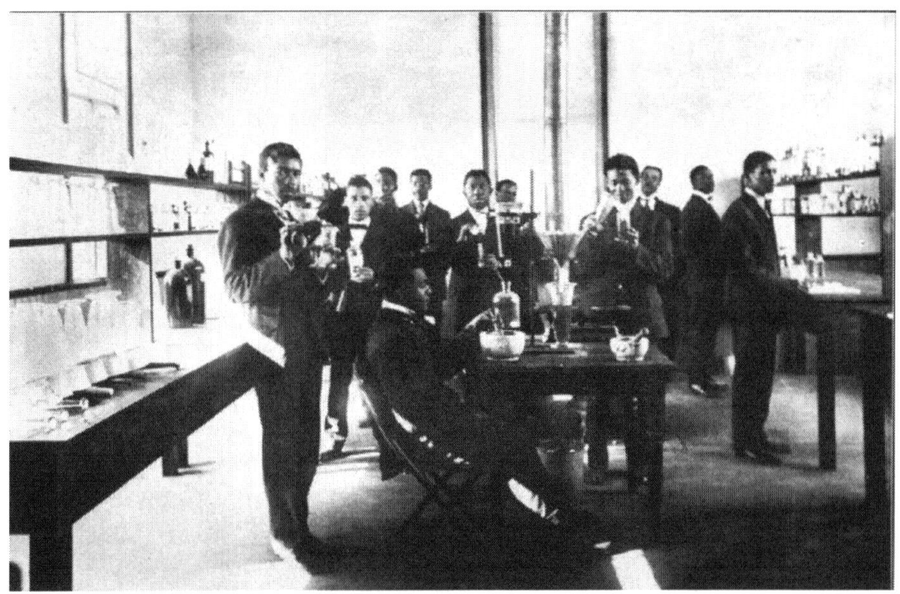

FIGURE 20. Pharmacy Students at Work in the Laboratory at Shaw Leonard School of Pharmacy.

(Source: Shaw University, *Twenty-Eight Annual Catalog of the Officers and Students of the Leonard School of Pharmacy, the Pharmaceutical Department of Shaw University*, [Raleigh, NC: Edwards & Broughton Printing Company, 1908].)

TABLE 10. Leonard School of Pharmacy Faculty: 1894–1912

NAME	RANK	COURSES	YEARS
William Simpson	Professor	Botany, Materia Medica, Pharmacy and Chemistry; Instructor, Compounding Medicine and Pharmacy Laboratory	1893–1906
Herbert B. Battle, Ph.D.	Professor	Medical and General Chemistry	1893–1896
H. K. Miller, M.S.	Professor	Medical and General Chemistry	1897–1898
J. M. Pickel, Ph.D.	Professor	Medical and General Chemistry	1898–1912
Charles B. Crowell, Ph.G.	Professor	Botany, Materia Medica, Pharmacy and Chemistry; Instructor, Compounding Medicine and Pharmacy Laboratory	1907–1910
Isaac A. Shade, Ph.G.	Assistant	Pharmacy Laboratory	1908–1910
Jno B. Watson, M.D., R.Ph.	Professor	Botany, Materia Medica, Pharmacy and Chemistry; Instructor, Compounding Medicine and Pharmacy Laboratory	1911–1912
C. L. Mallette, Ph.G.	Assistant	Pharmacy Laboratory	1910–1912

NAME	RANK	COURSES	YEARS
George T. Jones, Ph.G.	Demonstrator	Pharmacy	1911–1912

Source: Shaw University. *Fifteenth Annual Catalog of the Officers and Students of Leonard Medical School, For the Academic Year 1894-85,* (Raleigh, North Carolina: Shaw University, 1895); Shaw University. *Twenty-second Annual Catalog of the Officers and Teachers of the Leonard School of Pharmacy.* (Raleigh, North Carolina: Shaw University, 1912). https://archive.org/details/leonardschoolsof3219leon.

One of the most well-known amongst the two initial pharmacy faculty was *William Simpson*. He was Professor of Botany, Materia Medica, Pharmacy and Chemistry, and Instructor, Compounding Medicine and Pharmacy Laboratory.[226] Mr. Simpson was a pharmacist and teacher who grew up in New York, but moved with his family to Richmond, Virginia in 1844 and later to Raleigh, North Carolina. While working as a baker in his father's bakery business during the day, he studied in the evening as an apprentice in a local pharmacy (Ferguson Pharmacy) where he was able to later become a registered pharmacist in North Carolina. At the outbreak of the Civil War, Mr. Simpson volunteered for service in the Confederate Army with a Virginia regiment and was assigned as a pharmacist to a military hospital in Raleigh. After a brief duty of military service, not only did he work for a number of companies in the pharmaceutical business, including owning his own company, acquiring patents for several medicines, and publishing a pamphlet on fertilizer, he also became very active in professional associations in pharmacy.[227] He was a co-founder of the North Carolina Pharmaceutical Association (1880) and served as its President (1882–1883).[228]While teaching at the Leonard School of Pharmacy, Mr. Simpson became President of the American Pharmaceutical Association (1894–1895)[229] and served as Secretary-Treasurer of the North Carolina Board of Pharmacy (1881–1902).[230]

Dr. Herbert B. Battle was employed for a short period at Shaw University as the second initial faculty member and taught Medicinal and General Chemistry in the Leonard School of Pharmacy.[231] He was the son of the president (1876–1891) of the University of North Carolina (UNC). He received his Ph.D. in Chemistry at UNC in 1887.[232] While teaching at the School of Pharmacy, he was employed as the state chemist and director of the North Carolina Agricultural Experiment Station.[233] He left the School of Pharmacy around 1896 and became involved in a number of business ventures in Savannah, Georgia and later in Montgomery, Alabama. He was very active in his professional associations and became well known for his research work and as president with the Alabama Anthropological Society.[234]

Mr. H. K. Miller, M.S. taught at the School of Pharmacy from 1897–1898.[235] He replaced Dr. Battle and was the Assistant State Chemist at the North Carolina Agricultural Experiment Station.[236] He lectured on the chemical principles and process of importance to pharmacists.

Dr. J. M. Pickel, Ph.D. replaced H. K. Miller as the Professor of Medical and General Chemistry in the Leonard School of Pharmacy from 1898 to 1912. Dr. Pickel received his Ph.D. at the University of Berlin, Germany, and trained at Johns Hopkins University.[237]

Charles B. Crowell, Ph.C. replaced William Simpson as Professor of Botany, Materia Medica, Pharmacy and Chemistry. He received his pharmacy training and degree from the Maryland College of Pharmacy.[238]

Isaac A. Shade, Ph.G. (1908) and C. L. Mallette, Ph.G. (1910) were the first two African American pharmacists hired as part of the faculty and amongst the first in the U.S. to serve on a pharmacy school faculty. They were both Assistant in the Pharmacy Laboratory and graduates of the Leonard School of Pharmacy.[239]

Leonard School of Pharmacy started with very low numbers of students and faculty and only graduated one student in 1893 in their first class. The first Ph.G. degree was conferred upon *George P. Hart*, a student from Jacksonville, Florida.[240]

In the first eight years, from 1893–1900, the school's average enrollment was about six (6) students per year and graduated an average of three (3) students per year. (See **Table 11**.) By 1911, approximately 103 students had graduated from the Leonard School of Pharmacy. (See **Figures 21** and **22**.)

Although Shaw University had an admission policy that was open to women, it did not admit very many females into the professional pharmacy program.[241] *Pearl Rudolph Wassom* was the first African American female to receive the Ph.G. degree from the Leonard School of Pharmacy in 1897.[242] She was also one of only nine

African American females known to have received a pharmacy degree in the U.S. before 1900. (See **Table 12**.) The second of the only two females to graduate from the School of Pharmacy between 1897–1909, was *Shelley O. Brown,* Ph.G. (1909).[243]

TABLE 11. Pharmacy Graduates from the Pharmaceutical Department, Leonard School of Pharmacy: 1893–1911

Session	Graduates
1892–1893	1
1893–1894	6
1894–1895	5
1895–1896	2
1896–1897	8
1897–1898	1
1898–1899	—
1899–1900	6
1900–1901	1
1901–1902	3
1902–1903	5
1903–1904	7
1904–1905	6
1905–1906	13
1906–1907	5
1907–1908	7
1908–1909	12
1909–1910	9
1910–1911	6
Total	**103**

Source: Shaw University. *Twenty-second Annual Catalog of the Officers and Teachers of the Leonard School of Pharmacy.* The Pharmaceutical Department of Shaw University: Raleigh, North Carolina, 1912. https://archive.org/details/leonardschoolsof3219leon.

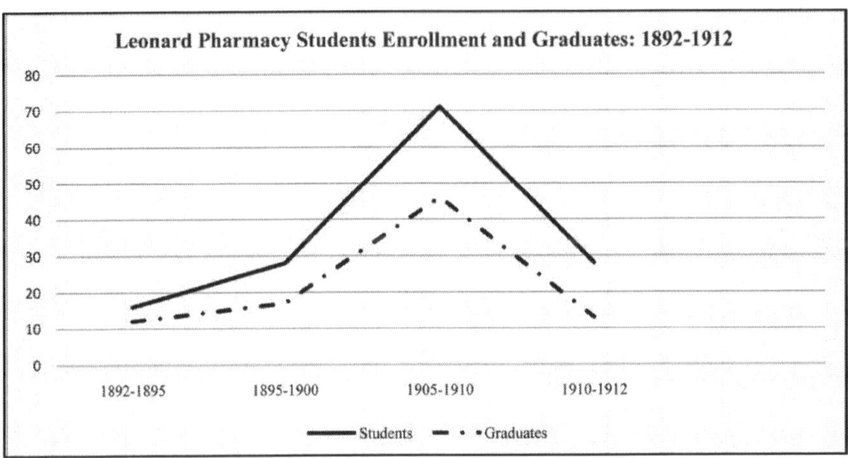

FIGURE 21. Leonard School of Pharmacy Students and Graduates: 1892–1911.

(Source: Shaw University, *Thirty-second Annual Catalog of the Officers and Students of the Leonard School of Pharmacy, The Pharmaceutical Department of Shaw University.* [Raleigh, NC: Edwards & Broughton Printing Company, 1912].)

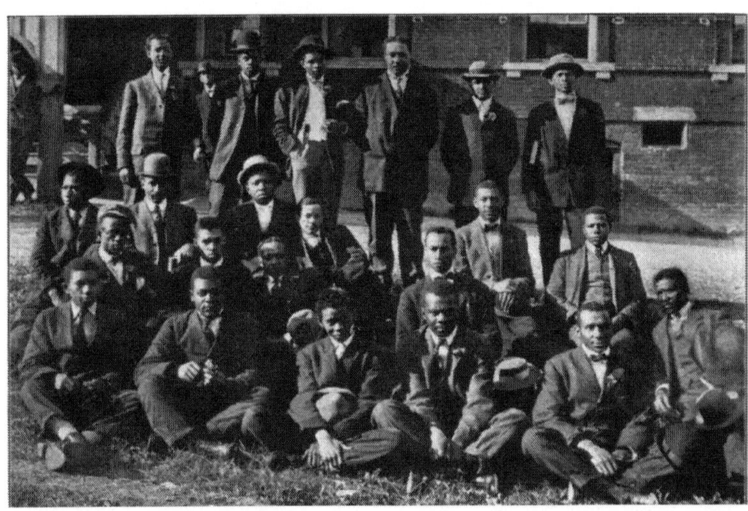

FIGURE 22. Leonard School of Pharmacy, Pharmacy Students, circa 1907.

(Source: *Eighteenth Annual Catalog of the Officers and Teachers of the Leonard School of Pharmacy, the Pharmaceutical Department of Shaw University, Raleigh, North Carolina,* 1908)

TABLE 12. African American Women Pharmacy Graduates Before 1900

Name	Degree*	Year	School
Ella A. Coleman	Ph.G.	1894	Meharry Pharmaceutical College
Matilda Lloyd	Ph.G.	1894	Meharry Pharmaceutical College
Margaret Miller	Ph.G.	1894	Meharry Pharmaceutical College
Susan Peters	Phar.G.	1895	Howard University Pharmaceutical College
Nannie B. Joyce	Ph.C.	1895	Meharry Pharmaceutical College
Pauline S. Marrow	Ph.C.	1896	Meharry Pharmaceutical College
Julia Pearl Hughes	Phar.D.	1897	Howard University Pharmaceutical College
Bellina S. Moore	Ph.C.	1897	Meharry Pharmaceutical College
Pearl R. Wassom	Ph.C.	1897	Shaw Leonard School of Pharmacy

Source: Meharry Medical College, "1935 Meharry Medical College Catalogue," *Meharry Medical College Archives*; Lamb, Daniel Smith, "Howard University Medical Department: A Historical, Biographical and Statistical Souvenir" (1900). *College of Medicine Publications.* Paper 1. http://dh.howard.edu/med_pub/1; *Eighth Annual Catalogue of the Officers and Students of Leonard School of Pharmacy, For the Academic Year Ending April 1, 1898* (Raleigh, NC: Shaw University, 1898).

*Ph.G.= *Graduate in Pharmacy*; Phar.G.= *Graduate in Pharmacy*; Ph.C.= *Pharmaceutical Chemist*; Phar.D.= *Doctor of Pharmacy*

Among the notable graduates of the Leonard School of Pharmacy was *James Edward Shepard*, who received the Ph.G. degree in 1894,[244] but chose to pursue a career in the ministry. He also received an honorary D.D. (Doctor of Divinity) degree from Muskingum College (OH) in 1910, the A.M. (Masters of Arts) degree from Selma University (AL) in 1912, and the honorary Litt.D. (Doctor of Literature) degree from Howard University in 1925.[245] (See **Figure 23**.) He became an internationally recognized businessman and educator, speaking and appearing in Europe, Africa, and the Caribbean

Islands throughout the early 1900s.[246] In 1909, he became the Founder and President of the North Carolina College for Negroes which continues today as North Carolina Central University (NCCU).[247] Because of his fundraising efforts, NCCU became one of the first state-supported liberal arts colleges for African Americans.[248] Other notable graduates of Leonard School of Pharmacy included *Robert McCants Harris*, Ph.G. (1914), owner of People's Drugs and President and Founder of the Union Mercantile Corporation of Waycross, GA.[249] (See **Figure 24**.)

Leonard School of Pharmacy produced some of the first African American pharmacists in the South. (See **Figure 25**.) By 1918, 131 African Americans had graduated from the School of Pharmacy.[250] (See **Table 13**.) More than 80% of the graduates remained in states throughout the South, and provided the pharmaceutical services needed to help address the health disparities so prevalent in the African American community. (See **Table 14**.)

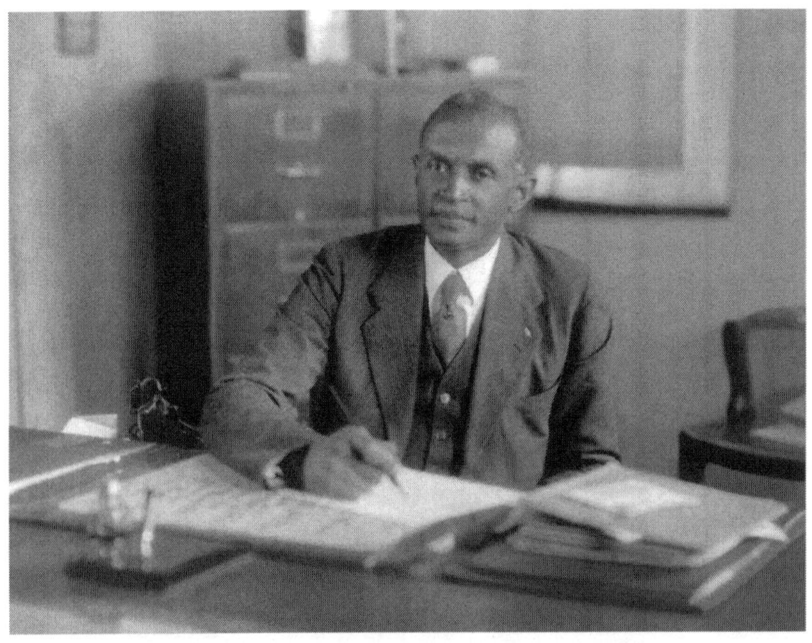

FIGURE 23. James Edward Shepard.

(Source: *Our Heritage: North Carolina Central University*, February 12, 2020, http://www.nccu.edu/we-are-nc-central/our-heritage)

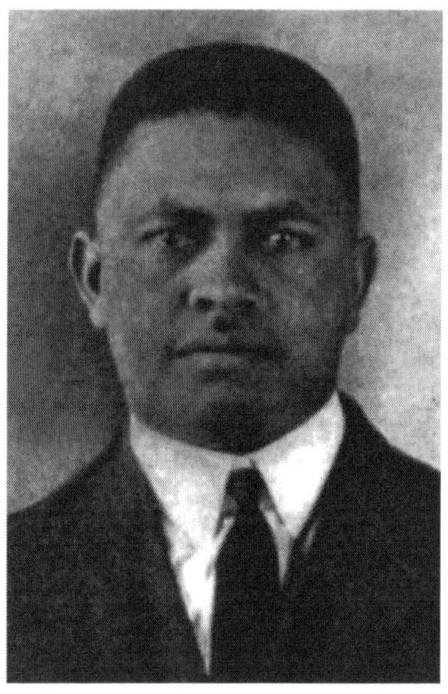

FIGURE 24. Robert McCants Harris.

(Source: *Who's Who in Colored America*, Yonkers-on-Hudson, N.Y.: C.E. Burckel, 232.)

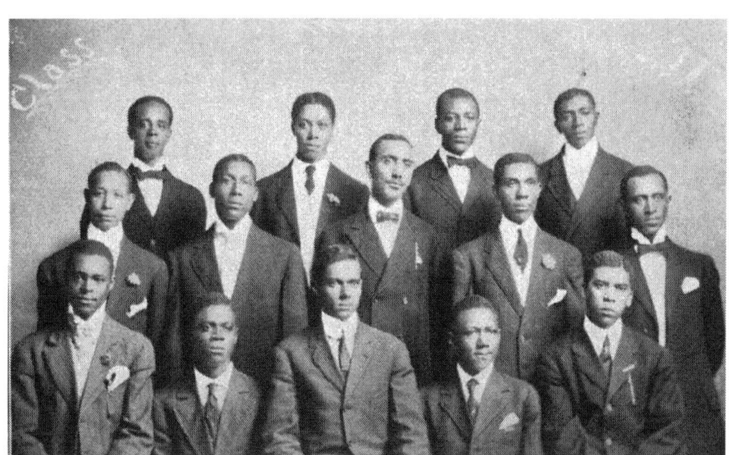

FIGURE 25. Leonard School of Pharmacy Class of 1911.

(Source: Shaw University, *Thirty-second Annual catalog of the Officers and Students of the Leonard School of Pharmacy, The Pharmaceutical Department of Shaw University.* [Raleigh, NC: Edwards & Broughton Printing Company, 1912].)

TABLE 13. Graduates of the Leonard School of Pharmacy: 1893–1911

CLASS	NAME	
1893	Hart, George P.	
1894	Alston, J. L. P	McNorton, R. C.
	Crews, C. F.	Perry, H. H.
	Eagles, J. L.	Shepard, James Edward
1895	Benson, J. M.	Newton, E. W.
	Dodson, J. A.	White, T. C.
	Hilton, P. H.	
1896	Bass, Eugene J.	
	Epps, Harry	
1897	Hasty, E. T.	McNair, W. L.
	Harris, John H.	Satterwhite, J. W.
	Merchant, E. C.	Vick, W. H.
	Morris, C. W.	Wassom, Pearl R.
1898	McCullough, J. H.	
1900	Jenkins, W. H.	Tatum, Huston H.
	Jones, W. A.	Thomas, W. E.
	Love, J. H.	Williams, H. E.
1901	Hall, Harry B.	
1902	Bass, Southall	
	Leboo, Prince	
	Scott, John	
1903	Andrews, R. E.	Roberts, J. N.
	Carter, E. R. , Jr. (M.D. '08)	Williston, F. C.
	Daniels, F. L.	
1904	Avant, F. W. (M.D. '08)	Jones, H. E.
	Douglass, J. D.	Shackelford, S. H., Jr.
	Eaton, J. H.	Watts, C. P.
	Fisher, H. A.	

CLASS	NAME	
1905	Fitzgerald, H. L.	Smith, J. T.
	Love, T. L., Jr.	Steward, C. H.
	McNair, F. W.	Tate, S. M.
1906	Corbin. H.	Kennedy, H. P., Jr.
	Dorsey, J. S.	Macbeth, W. L.
	Ellison, F. Y.	Neal, S.
	Harris, R. M.	Porter, William M.
	Hayley, W. E.	Shade, Isaac A.
	Holland, T. C.	Yancey, D. C.
	Holliday, C. C.	
1907	Beaman, W. Troy	Fuller, John W.
	Bowles, Allen M.	Patterson James H., Jr.
	Drake, Thomas C.	
1908	Bryant, Franke E.	Rogers, W. Thomas
	Grigg, H. B.	Williams, Thos. J
	Henderson, A. J.	Yancey, L. A.
	Robinson, J. M.	
1909	Blue, Henry C.	Moseley, Hiram A. J.
	Brown, Shelley O.	Riley, George T.
	Burwell, L. Gladstone	Sharp, Boston, C.
	Jackson, Henry H.	Smith, William A.
	Jones, George T.	Webb, James B.
	Mallette, Charles L.	Whitehead, Henry J.
1910	Brown, Thomas J.	Harris, John. T.
	Bornette, Baker J.	Pearson, John W.
	Coleman, William P.	Perry, Dallas
	Eaton, Benjamin H.	Williams, Roger A.
	Gaylord, Felton C.	
1911	Bridgeford, William V.	Graham, James J.
	Dunston, C. William	Hairston, Jacob W.
	Frederick, Robert James	Hamlin, James T.

Source: *Twenty-second Annual Catalog of the Officers and Teachers of the Leonard School of Pharmacy, the Pharmaceutical Department of Shaw University. For the Academic Year Ending May thirty-first Nineteen Hundred and Twelve,* (Raleigh, NC: Shaw University, 1912)

TABLE 14. Geographical Distribution of Shaw Leonard School of Pharmacy Graduates After Graduation: 1893–1911

State	Number (%)
Alabama	5 (5)
District of Columbia	1 (1)
Georgia	3 (2.9)
Illinois	3 (2.9)
Kentucky	2 (1.9)
Louisiana	1 (1)
Massachusetts	1 (1)
Missouri	2 (1.9)
New Jersey	1 (1)
North Carolina	50 (49)
Pennsylvania	2 (1.9)
South Carolina	9 (8.8)
Tennessee	3 (2.9)
Texas	2 (1.9)
Virginia	12 (11.8)
West Virginia	5 (5)

Sources: *Twenty-second Annual Catalog of the Officers and Teachers of the Leonard School of Pharmacy, The Pharmaceutical Department of Shaw University*, (Raleigh, NC: Shaw University, 1912).

There were several factors associated with the closing of the Shaw University medical and pharmacy schools, as well as the other professional degree programs. One key factor was the death of Dr. Henry Tupper in 1893.[251] After his passing, his predecessor was rumored to not have the same passion, enthusiasm, and vision for the school.[252] Dr. Charles F. Meserve, LLD succeeded Dr. Henry Tupper and was the President of the University up until the closing of the pharmacy and medical schools.[253] Other factors included the termination of annual financial appropriations to the University by the American Baptist Home Mission Society.[254] There was also a national movement to reform medical education in the United States and Canada,[255] which made it difficult for the Medical School to keep up with the changing medical education standards. Racism, financial controversies, and differences in philosophy of the religious mission of the school all added to the challenges.[256] In 1914, the financial difficulties forced the Medical School to close. Since the pharmacy school was so closely linked to the School of Medicine, its closing followed in 1918.

4 University of West Tennessee College of Pharmacy

John E. Clark

The state of Tennessee was unique in that it was the only state to provide two pharmacy education programs for African Americans after U.S. Civil War. The most well-known of the Tennessee programs is Meharry Pharmaceutical College. The other school was the University of West Tennessee (UWT) College of Pharmacy. There is reason to suspect the Chattanooga National Medical College in Chattanooga, Tennessee might have been the third since there was some indication in its charter of the intent to hire faculty to teach pharmacy, but the College closed after four years and never expanded its program beyond the teaching of medical students.[257]

The University of West Tennessee (UWT) was co-founded in 1900 by Dr. Miles Vandahurst Lynk and his wife, Beebe Steven Lynk, in Jackson, Tennessee. (See **Figure 26**.) Dr. Lynk was a 1891 graduate of the Meharry Medical College.[258] He was the co-founder of the National Medical Association (the black counterpart to the American Medical Association).[259] The organization was originally formed at the Cotton States and International Exposition of 1895 in Atlanta, Georgia.[260] The name was officially changed to the National Medical Association a few years later.[261]

Dr. Lynk was the editor and publisher of the first African American medical journal, *The Medical and Surgical Observer.*[262] (See **Figure 27**.) He also started his own magazine (*Lynk's Magazine*),[263] publishing company,[264] and wrote three books, including his autobiography, entitled *Sixty Years of Medicine or the Life and Times of Dr. Miles V. Lynk, an Autobiography* (1951).[265]

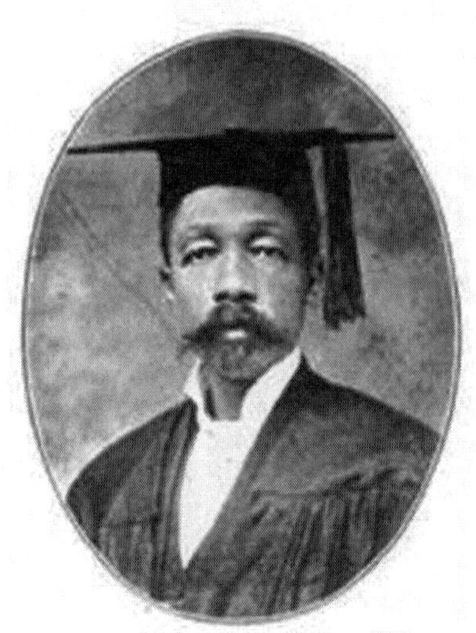

FIGURE 26: Miles V. Lynk.

(Source: "Miles Vandahurst Lynk," *Wikipedia, The Free Encyclopedia,* https://en.wikipedia.org/w/index.php?title=Miles_Vandahurst_Lynk&oldid=864813912 (accessed June 11, 2020).

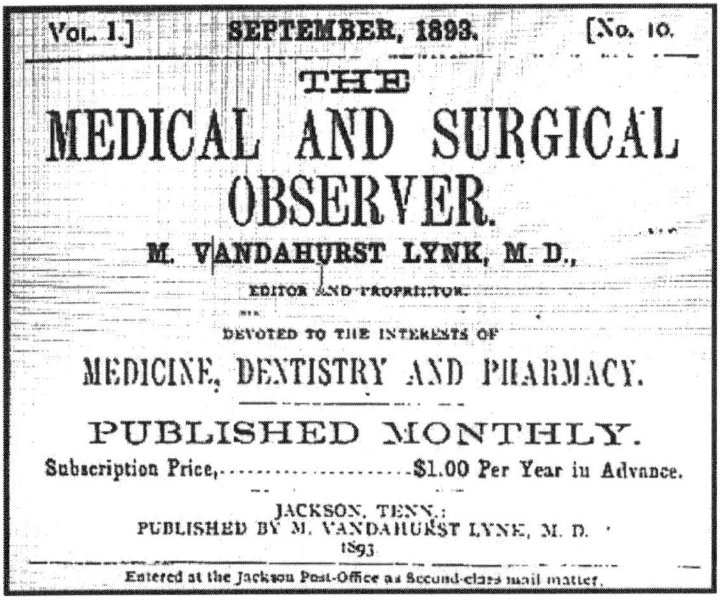

VOL. 1.] SEPTEMBER, 1893. [No. 10.

THE

MEDICAL AND SURGICAL OBSERVER.

M. VANDAHURST LYNK, M. D.,

EDITOR AND PROPRIETOR.

DEVOTED TO THE INTERESTS OF

MEDICINE, DENTISTRY AND PHARMACY.

PUBLISHED MONTHLY.

Subscription Price,....................$1.00 Per Year in Advance.

JACKSON, TENN.:
PUBLISHED BY M. VANDAHURST LYNK, M. D.
1893

Entered at the Jackson Post-Office as Second-class mail matter.

FIGURE 27. *J Natl Med Assoc.* 1996 Feb; 88(2): 115-22.

For several years, Dr. Lynk had a vision of starting a health science school of higher education because of a shortage of African American physicians in the South and because white medical schools restricted the admission and training of African Americans. He approached several prominent gentlemen and friends in the city of Jackson and presented his idea. The men included: Reverend Robert E. Hart, pastor of the C.M.E. Church; Mr. James H. Trimble, postman and mail carrier; Drs. John L. Light and Samuel H. Broome. They got together and applied to the state of Tennessee, and were granted articles of incorporation on December 20, 1900 to start the school that became the University of West Tennessee.[266]The UWT did not receive its charter by the State of Tennessee until November 22, 1901. Although the school was generally thought of as a proprietary, for-profit school, it was advertised in the Annual Announcements as being established by the state of Tennessee under its charter for: "The general welfare of society, not individual profit, … , and hence the members are not stockholders in the legal sense of the term, and no dividends or profits shall be divided among the members."[267] The income, resources, and equipment were intended to be dedicated for the benefit of educating African Americans. Dr. Lynk's vision was to create a school for the training of physicians and surgeons in addition to providing professional training opportunities in dentistry, pharmacy, nursing, and law.

The principal organizers and administrators of the school programs were Dr. Mile V. Lynk, Dr. Samuel Henry Broome, and Mrs. Beebe Stevens Lynk. They were responsible for the development of the curriculum, recruitment of faculty, development of the training facilities and sites, and acquiring the space for the classes and training. Because there were no endowments, government subsidies, student loans, or financial support from religious organizations, the school also began with significant financial problems and had to constantly look for alternative ways for raising money. Mrs. Lynk and her husband are reported to have mortgaged their home and used the money to purchase the building and the lot for the university, as well as an addition of a third floor to the building and needed merchandise and equipment.[268] (See **Figure 28**.)

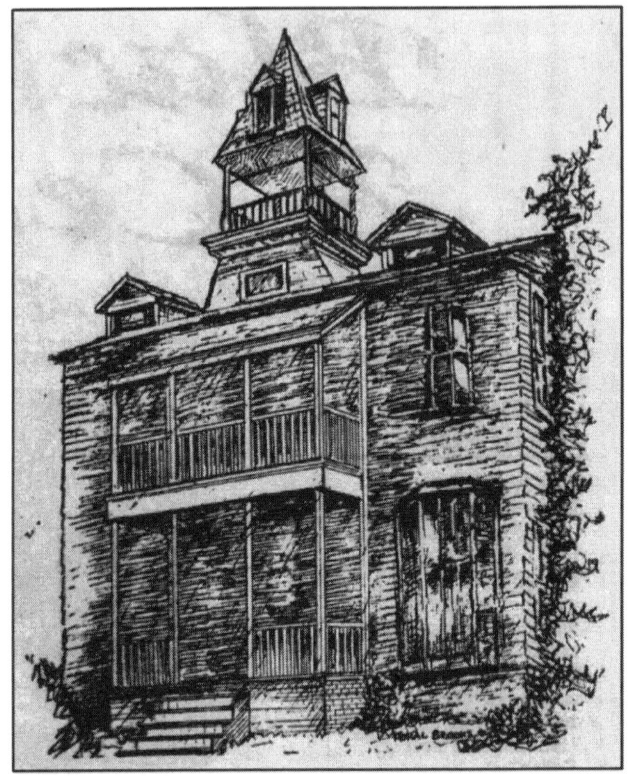

FIGURE 28. Artist impression of the University of West Tennessee Building, 1907.

(Source: Ronal Brooks, *The Jackson Sun*, February 18, 1994, 32)

The pharmacy program started in 1901 as a department of the University of West Tennessee (UWT). Initially, it was a two-year program, and became a three-year program in 1906 with each session continuing for 26 weeks.[269] (See **Table 15**.) All applicants for admission had to be: (1) at least 18 years of age; (2) of good moral character; (3) able to satisfactorily pass an entrance examination in English, and; (4) have a working knowledge of the fundamentals of Latin and Physics.[270] The school had an open admission policy regardless of race, gender, state, or country. The school admitted male and female students from all over the U.S. and six foreign countries. Students paid a tuition fee of $30.00 per session.

TABLE 15. University of West Tennessee College of Pharmacy Courses: 1909–1910

First Year
• Chemistry • Materia Medica • Pharmacy • Medical Latin • Work in Chemical and Pharmaceutic Laboratories
Second Year
• Materia Medica • Pharmacy • Qualitative Analysis • Botany • Toxicology • Medical Chemistry • Laboratory Work
Third Year
• Volumetric and Gravimetric Analysis • Milk and Water Analysis • Microscopy • Hygiene • Pharmaceutic Arithmetic • Urinalysis • Synthetic Chemistry • Pharmacy

Source: University of West Tennessee, *Catalogue for the Session of 1909-10: Announcement for the Session of 1910-11* (Memphis, TN: University of West Tennessee, 1911).

Requirements for graduation were like other schools of this time. The candidate:

1. Had to be at least twenty-one years of age, and of good moral character;
2. Had to have attended at least three sessions of pharmaceutical courses, of not less than 24 weeks each, the last of which must have been at the UWT;
3. Must have satisfactorily passed written examinations in all branches of the course, including the outline of Bible history and its doctrine; and
4. Performed the required number of hours of laboratory work in the practice of pharmacy.

Once all requirements were met, the Pharmaceutical Chemist (Ph.C.) degree was awarded.[271]

The Pharmacy Department's inaugural class, in 1901, was comprised of four students.[272] They all graduated in 1903 with the Ph.C. degree. In 1907, Dr. Lynk moved the school to 1190 South Phillips Place in Memphis, and by then had graduated 16 physicians, one dentist, four pharmacists, and five lawyers.[273] During the early 1900s, Memphis had become a very attractive city for African American professionals. One of the largest concentrations of black practicing physicians and other medical professionals in the State of Tennessee could be found in Memphis. Most of the physicians were trained at Meharry Medical College. Some of the well-known faculty that supported the UWT Medical College and the Pharmacy Department included:

- Dr. Francis M. Kneeland, one of the first black female physicians in Memphis;
- Dr. Cleveland A. Terrell and his nephew, Dr. L.O. Patterson, co-founded the Terrell-Patterson Infirmary and the Jane Terrell Memorial Hospital, facilities where the medical and nursing students from UWT trained; and

- Dr. Jacob C. Hairston, who trained Dr. Lynk as an apprentice and later established the Hairston Hospital, which was also used for the training of students.[274]

After moving to Memphis, the UWT Medical School faculty increased in numbers and in the specialty background of various practitioners and in the number of faculty teaching in the Pharmacy Department. The pharmacy faculty was primarily medical physicians, both black and white.[275] Two of the small faculty of five had degrees in the pharmaceutical sciences. Mr. George R. Jackson, who received his Ph.G. from the University of Michigan (1892) and was the first black pharmacist in Memphis,[276] joined the faculty as Professor of Theoretical and Practical Pharmacy.[277] Mrs. Beebe Steven Lynk, who received her Pharmaceutical Chemist (Ph.C.) degree from the UWT Department of Pharmacy (1903), joined the faculty as Professor of Chemistry and Pharmacy and thus became one of the first African American women in the U.S. to teach in a pharmacy and medical program.

At the start of the 1909 session, the pharmacy program was referred to as the College of Pharmacy in the official annual catalogues and announcements.[278] There were five students in the 1909 class.[279] The faculty included:

- Miles V. Lynk, M.D. (Professor of *Materia Medica*, Botany and Microscopy)
- Beebe S. Lynk, Ph.C. (Professor of Chemistry)
- J. B. Freeland, B.S. (Chemical Laboratory)
- Nathaniel H.C. Henderson, M.D. (Professor of Physiology and Hygiene)

Dr. Miles Lynk served as President and Dean of the Medical College and did the bulk of the teaching in all branches of the university, including the law school. Beebe Stevens Lynk was the primary faculty member responsible for teaching and organizing the courses in the UWT pharmacy program. In the 1923 graduation class photo (see **Figure 29**), she is listed as Dean of the University of West Tennessee (UWT).[280] It appears that with this appointment, Beebe Stevens Lynk became the first African American female in the nation that graduated from a pharmacy degree program to serve as Dean of a health science institution.[281]

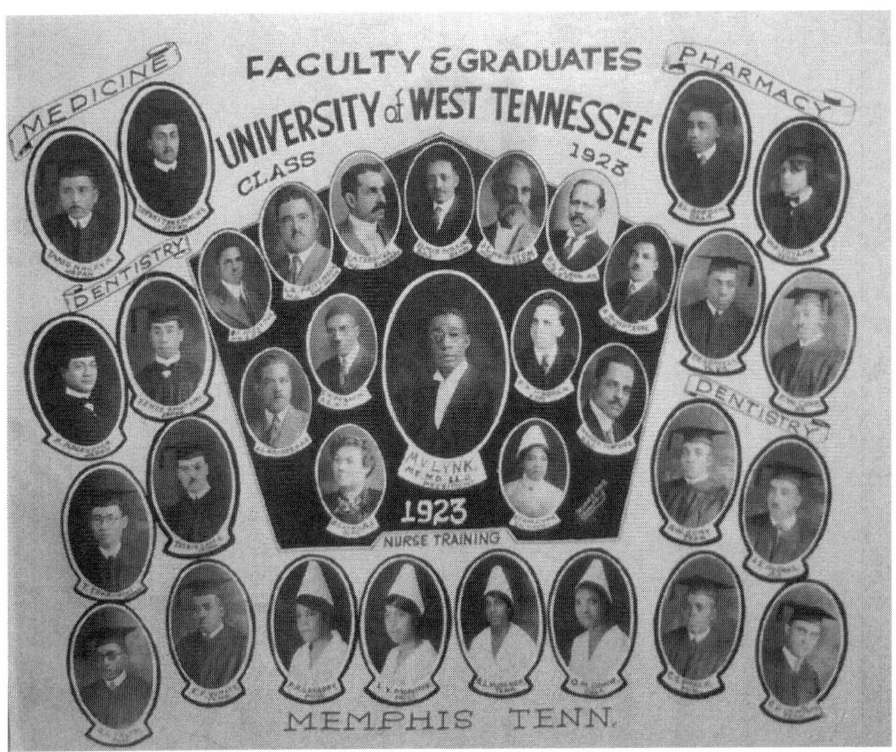

FIGURE 29. University of West Tennessee Class of 1923.

(Source: Ernestine Lovelle Jenkins. *Faculty and Graduates University of West Tennessee, Class of 1923.* In *Images of America: African Americans in Memphis,* [Charleston, SC: Arcadia Publishing, 2009], 42.)

Like other African American healthcare schools, UWT suffered financial constraints from the time it opened. In efforts to raise money to sustain the school, Dr. Lynk formed the UWT Vandahurst Musical Quartette, which was made up of faculty and students.[282] In 1916, the singers went on tour through the states of Alabama and Georgia and performed to packed audiences at various churches and theaters around Birmingham and Atlanta. Although Dr. Lynk toured with the singers, it is uncertain whether he sang with the group. The company was composed of Mrs. Beebe Stevens Lynk, soprano; Mrs. J.A. Brady, alto and reader; H.W. Williamson, tenor; and M.R. McWhorton, bass. Miss B. G. Stevens, coloratura soprano, was the soloist.[283]

In 1909, the school was inspected by Abraham Flexner of the Carnegie Foundation and received a less than favorable assessment. The Report by Flexner casted doubt on the quality of equipment, resources, facilities, teaching, and overall integrity of the school. It became even more difficult to maintain high educational standards because of the cost imposed during this intense period. In 1912, only 1 out of 14 applicants from UWT College of Medicine passed the state licensing examination.[284] The reputation of the school deteriorated such that some state licensing boards would not recognize the diploma of the Medical College graduates.[285] By 1916, the enrollment started to decline drastically. With only a grim chance of recovering, Dr. Lynk and his administration decided to close the school.[286] By the time the school closed in 1923, approximately 155 physicians and many other early black health professionals in Memphis had received training at the UWT.[287]

The College of Pharmacy was active for more than 20 years. The total number of pharmacists that graduated from UWT is not known. Detailed records of the school appear to have been lost or destroyed. The pharmacy department started with 4 students in the first class. It does not appear that the numbers exceeded 6 students per class. There were 4 graduates identified in the 1903 class,[288] 5 in the 1910 class,[289] 3 in the 1911 class, and 4 in the 1923 class.[290] (See **Table 16**.). Not much is reported about their careers as pharmacists after graduation.

TABLE 16. Graduates of the University of West Tennessee College of Pharmacy

CLASS	NAME
1903	Anderson, T. L.
	Lynk, Beebe Steven
	Steven, Willie Ann
	Woodson, J. H.
1910	Davis, C. T.
	Flood, H. G.
	Gunn, J. B.
	Powell, B. S.
	Wiley, H. L.
1923	Barber, R. L.
	Cook, F. W.
	Gravely, T. R.
	Taylor, W. E.

The most well-known of the graduates from the UWT pharmacy program is Mrs. Beebe Stevens Lynk. In 1900, she became the first known African American woman to co-establish a health science school of higher learning when she and her husband established the University of West Tennessee and began offering degrees in medicine, dentistry, pharmacy, and nursing. Prior to her marriage, she had graduated from Lane College in Jackson, Tennessee in 1892 and worked for several years as a schoolteacher. She had two brothers, Albert Stevens, and Jackson Stevens, and four sisters, Willie Ann Stevens, Agnes Eudora Stevens, Eleanor Stevens, and Blanche Stevens. When she decided to enter the UWT Pharmacy Department, her sister Willie Ann Stevens joined her. They both graduated with the Ph.C. degree in 1903. It appears that neither of the two women became registered pharmacists. After graduation, her sister, Willie Ann Stevens, went to work as a schoolteacher in the Tipton County, Tennessee, public school district along with her younger sister, Blanche Stevens. At the same time, Beebe Stevens Lynk became one of the first African American women to serve on a faculty of a health science school when she was appointed Professor of Chemistry and Pharmacy at UWT. She was active in the Colored Women's Clubs and served as chapter Treasurer of the Tennessee Federation of Colored Women Clubs. She also had an interest in hair and beauty products for African American women. With her pharmaceutical chemistry background, she developed her own recipes for cold and vanishing creams, shampoos, lotions, skin beaching, and hair growth products. Her recipes were provided in a book she published entitled *A Complete Course in Hair Straightening and Beauty Culture* (Memphis, TN: 20th Century Art Company, 1919).

The two men in the same class (1903) were able to work in pharmacy after graduation. Mr. T. L. Anderson moved to Clearwater, Oklahoma, and Mr. John H. Woodson moved to Gulfport, Mississippi, where they both were able to establish themselves as pharmacists.

5 New Orleans University College of Pharmacy

John E. Clark, Diane S. Allen-Gipson

At the end of the Civil War, New Orleans became one of those cities like others in the south where freed slaves congregated upon leaving the confines of the plantations. Like other large cities in the south, New Orleans faced a healthcare and economic crisis due to a lack of basic health services and jobs to accommodate the newly emancipated slaves. In July 1869, the Freedman's Aid Society of the Methodist Episcopal Church founded the New Orleans University (originally named the Union Normal School) to meet the educational and healthcare needs of the African American population. The institution initially provided courses at the elementary, secondary, collegiate and professional education levels for African Americans. In 1889, the university opened the Medical College of New Orleans University, in a new building at the corner of Canal and Robertson Streets, near the center of the city. In 1901, the Medical Department was named Flint Medical College of New Orleans University in honor of Mr. John D. Flint for his generous endowment.[291] The purpose of the Department was to produce African American doctors and to facilitate organized healthcare for the black community in and around the city of New Orleans. The program also provided professional education for black men and women in nursing and pharmacy.[292]

In September 1900, the New Orleans University College of Pharmacy of Flint Medical College opened. When it opened, there was another pharmacy program with a similar name in New Orleans, the New Orleans College of Pharmacy, a white school that was incorporated in 1900 by its founder, Dr. Philip Asher.[293] From the beginning, Dr. Asher chose to affiliate with Loyola University of New Orleans. In 1913, Loyola University acquired the New Orleans College of Pharmacy, and completely merged by 1919 as the Loyola University College of Pharmacy.[294] As other pharmacy schools opened in Louisiana, competition increased, and the Loyola College of Pharmacy enrollment began to decline. Enrollment reached a low in the 1957–58 school year. While carrying a 5-year consecutive average deficit of $1,200 per student, the administration decided to close the Loyola University College of Pharmacy in 1965.[295]

The New Orleans University College of Pharmacy of the Flint Medical College was a co-educational program whose educational focus was to produce African American pharmacists. The College of Pharmacy and the entire university had an open admission policy, which was slightly different from that of Loyola University. Loyola University was considered co-educational and the College of Pharmacy continued to enroll female students, even though they weren't admitted as full-time Loyola University liberal arts undergraduates until the 1950s.[296] In some of their earlier catalogues, the New Orleans University College of Pharmacy of Flint Medical College was promoted as being the only such school in the South that was opened to all regardless of race, religion, and gender.[297] Women were admitted under the same terms, conditions, and criteria as men. In most lecture halls, public clinics, and laboratories, women attended the classes and course activities alongside men.[298]

The requirements for admission were like those of the Medical College. To attend the College of Pharmacy, the candidates: (1) had to have a thorough knowledge of English grammar, composition, and rhetoric, as well as mathematics, geometry, elementary physics, and United States History; and (2) an understanding of Latin, covering at least one book of Caesar's Commentaries.[299]

The pharmacy curriculum was extended over three sessions of 28 weeks each year. Much of the course activity involved laboratory work in compounding, chemistry, and preparation of drug products. The tuition fee was $40.00 per session and classes were offered in the day and at night for working students.[300] (See **Table 17**.)

TABLE 17. New Orleans University College of Pharmacy Courses: 1900–1901

First Year
• Botany • Chemistry • Materia Medica • Pharmacy • Medical Latin • Elements of Physics • Laboratory Work
Second Year
• Materia Medica • Pharmacy • Analytical Chemistry • Pharmacognosy • Toxicology • Laboratory Work
Third Year
• Medical and Pharmaceutical Chemistry • Microscopy • Laboratory Work • Pharmacy

Source: *Year Book of the New Orleans University, 1900 – 1901* (New Orleans, LA: Flint Medical College, 1901).

To graduate, the candidates: (1) had to be at least 21 years of age, of good moral character; (2) must have attended three sessions of pharmaceutical course work; (3) must have satisfactorily passed examination in all the course work; and (4) be mentally and morally fit for the assumption of the role of a pharmacist. Students meeting all requirements were awarded the Pharmaceutical Chemist (Ph.C.) degree.[301] In 1911, the College started awarding the Graduate in Pharmacy (Ph.G.) degree, which continued up until the school's closing.[302]

The initial enrollment in the College of Pharmacy in 1900 included three students:[303]

1. Miss Lucy Gonzales (Bocas del Toro, Colombia, South America)
2. Miss Camille Green (New Orleans, LA)
3. Mr. James D. Weathers (Woodville, MS)

When the first class graduated in 1903, it included five students, three men and two women, and only one student from the inaugural class.[304] Miss Camille O. Green was one of the women in the inaugural class.[305] Miss Green and classmate Minnie C. Moore became the first known African American female graduates of a pharmacy school program in the state of Louisiana.[306] Minnie Moore is later listed in the 1910 U.S. Census as operating her own drugstore in Jackson, Mississippi.[307] Camille Green joined the faculty in the College of Pharmacy after graduation, serving as Professor of Pharmacy from 1903 to 1908. With her appointment, Camille Green became one of the first African American female faculty members of a College of Pharmacy. Her appointment occurred the same year as Beebe Stevens Lynk's. The College of Pharmacy faculty was comprised of primarily physicians from the medicine department and at least five pharmacy degree faculty throughout the duration of the program. Camille Green was the only female faculty member with a pharmacy degree who taught in the New Orleans University College of Pharmacy. (See **Table 18**.)

Camille O. Green married Thomas Herman Mims on July 18, 1906, a physician she met when he was a medical student attending the Flint Medical College. They moved to Philadelphia in 1909 where she went back to pharmacy school at Temple University and graduated with her second pharmacy degree (Ph.G.) in 1911. In 1912, she and her husband moved back to New Orleans where he set up his medical practice and she established herself as a practicing pharmacist.[308]

TABLE 18. New Orleans University Flint Medical College of Pharmacy Faculty: 1900–1914

NAME	RANK	COURSES	YEAR
H. J. Clements, M.S., M.D.	Dean/Professor	Chemistry and Materia Medica	1900–1901
Aristide R. DeJoie, Ph.C	Professor	Pharmacy	1900–1913
J. Robert Bean	Instructor	Chemistry	1900–1901
E. L. Hamilton	Instructor	Medical Latin	1900–1901
Camille O. Green-Mims, Ph.C.	Professor	Pharmacy	1903–1908
Thaddeus Taylor, A.B.	Instructor	Medical Latin	1904–1905
W. H. Harrison, M.S., M.D.	Professor	Materia Medica	1904–1908
Valcour A. Chapman, Ph.C.	Instructor	Pharmacy	1906–1912
H. W. Cummings, B.S.	Professor	Chemistry, Physics	1906–1908
R. T. Fuller, M.D.	Dean/Professor	Pharmacology	1911–1914
Edward F. Lopez, Phar.D.	Professor	Pharmacy	1911–1914
G. B. Kramer, M.D.	Professor	Chemistry, Bacteriology, Physics	1911–1914
L. T. Burbridge, M.D.	Professor	Materia Medica and Therapeutics	1911–1914
J. A. Hardin, M.D.	Professor	Toxicology	1911–1914
Rives Fredricks, M.D.	Professor	Physiology	1911–1913
Joseph M. Nelson, Ph.G.	Professor	Commercial Pharmacy	1911–1912
R. Vining, M.D.	Professor	Therapeutics	1912–1914

Source: *Tan and Blue Catalogue Edition, New Orleans University 1913-1914* (New Orleans, LA: E. T. Harvey & Son Printers, 1914).

Aristide Romar Dejoie, Ph.C. was one of the inaugural pharmacy faculty members who taught in the College of Pharmacy from 1900 to 1913. He was a very active civic, political, and business leader during the Reconstruction Period in Louisiana. His accomplishments included being elected an Assessor in Orleans Parish and serving on the World Cotton Centennial Exposition Commission.[309] He also served on the State Central Executive Committee of the Republican Party of Louisiana, which was headed by P. B. S. Pinchback,[310] and on several other special committees of the Louisiana House of Representatives.[311] Dejoie was a 1899 graduate of the Meharry Pharmaceutical College and was associated with the pharmacy program up until its closing.[312]

Other pharmacy-trained faculty of the College of Pharmacy included: Valcour A. Chapman, Ph.C. (Flint, 1907), Edward F. Lopez, Phar.D., and Joseph N. Nelson, Ph.G. (Flint, 1909). Valcour Chapman received the Ph.C. degree from the Flint Medical College Pharmacy Department in 1907. He was a clergyman from St. Charles Parish, Louisiana. He was ordained as a minister (M.E.) in 1883 and served as member of the Louisiana Conference. He was also a presiding elder of the New Orleans South District of the Louisiana Conference from 1897 to 1899 and district superintendent in 1910. He taught in the public-school system for 10 years and in the Flint Medical College of Pharmacy from 1907–1911.[313]

The Dean of the College of Medicine, H. J. Clements, M.S., M.D., also served as the founding Dean of the College of Pharmacy. Two other Deans, Dr. A. D. Bush, M.D. (1907–1911) and Dr. Ray T. Fuller, M.D. (1911–1914), succeeded Dr. Clements as head of both the College of Medicine and College of Pharmacy up until its closing.

The Flint Medical College closed in 1911 under financial constraints that it had been dealing with since its beginning. A major portion of the funding for the school came from the Freedmen's Aid Society of the Methodist Episcopal Church. One of the goals of the Freedmen's Aid Society was to establish and maintain educational institutions in the South for the black community.[314] Although impeded by racial hostility among the Southern white community for many years, the Society consistently had two fundamental and related difficulties to overcome: (1) the scarcity of the financial resources upon which it could draw, and (2) the fragmentation of American

Methodism at the time, which led to small amounts of benevolent contributions from Southern congregations (versus Northern). Very unstable financial conditions of the Society evolved, which became the primary cause of the chronic financial problem that plagued the medical department at the New Orleans University from the beginning.[315] When the medical department was charted to open in 1873, it did not open until 1877 because of inadequate funds. A new financial plan was implemented to sustain the medical program in the 1878–79 school term, but it failed, and the medical department was closed in 1881. After further discussion and planning, the new medical department was reintroduced in 1889 and offered a three-year course of study, higher admission standards and graduation requirements. From 1889 until 1897, the medical department grew despite racial and financial impediments. The curriculum expanded to a four-year course of study, the faculty increased in size, buildings were renovated to accommodate the education and training of new students, and the annual budget increased.[316]

When the medical college seemed to be making progress, it became a subject of the report of the Carnegie Foundation for the Advancement of Teaching. In the 1910 Flexner report, the Flint Medical College was one of five out of seven historically black medical colleges recommended to be closed because of inadequate training and facilities to meet current standards of medical education.[317] Shortly thereafter, the Flint Medical College closed in 1911. The College of Pharmacy and Nurse Training School continued for a few years longer. By 1913, the College of Pharmacy had graduated approximately 60 African American pharmacists. (See **Table 19** and **Table 20**.) Most of the pharmacy graduates (59%) remained in the South, primarily in the State of Louisiana (see **Table 21**), and thus filled a void for pharmaceutical healthcare in the African American community that was sorely needed in the South. (See **Figure 30**.)

TABLE 19. Pharmacy Graduates from the New Orleans College of Pharmacy: 1900–1914

Session	New Students Enrolled	Total Graduates
1900–1901	3	0
1901–1902	3	0
1902–1903	—	5
1903–1904	9	1
1904–1905	13	1
1905–1906	20	2
1906–1907	22	8
1907–1908	23	3
1908–1909	—	4
1909–1910	—	10
1910–1911	10	7
1911–1912	24	8
1912–1913	24	3
1913–1914	26	8
Total	**129**	**60**

Sources: New Orleans University, *Tan and Blue Annual Catalogue Edition, New Orleans University 1913-1914.* E.T. Harvey & Son: New Orleans, LA, 1914, accessed January 10, 2016, http://hdl.handle.net/2027/uiuo.ark:/13960/t7dr4fc96

TABLE 20. Graduates of the New Orleans College of Pharmacy for Flint Medical College: 1903–1914

CLASS	NAME	
1903	Greene, Camille O.	
	Major, Joseph E.	
	Moore, Minnie C.	
	Porter, Percy W.	
	Watts, Perry W.	
1904	Taylor Henry	
1905	Christophe, W. R.	
1906	Peters, James E.	
	Johnson, Dan J.	
1907	Chapman, Valcour	Harlan, Q. Z
	Dejoie, Joseph J.	Newman, Gershon
	Duncan, Stephen J.	Pemilton, Clarence A.
	Gair, James	Landry, E. P.
1908	Baumann, Albert	
	Morrell, David C.	
	Peete, Thomas H.	
1909	Hall, James C.	
	Nelson, Joseph	
	Waddell, Charles	
	Miller, Theodore L.	
1910	Blanchet, Louis A.	Maurice, Raoul J.
	Brazier, J. Sidney	Overton, Lebanon
	Barrois, Robert U.	Peters, Preston B.
	Johnson, Arthur C.	Speight, Virginia
	Kyle, William	Ware, Mattic S.
1911	Donaldson, Mary A.	Thomas, G. B.
	Dright, Carrie E.	Walker, Arthur R.

CLASS	NAME	
1911	Griffin, Wade E.	Worsham, Oscar B.
	Jamison, Mary E.	
1912	Dyson, Hosea E.	Lee, Abijah O.
	Fleming, Augustus C.	Polkington, Jas. R.
	Gowen, Frank A.	Stewart, Bush, Jr.
	Johnson, August J.	Shallowhorn, Lucille J.
1913	Dauphiune, Mabel	
	Hudson, Louis C.	
	Tarver, Uriah I.	
1914	Bucksell, Louis P.	Segue, R. Ernest
	Gray, Sidney A.	Taper, Albert J.
	Harris, William	Vesha, Leo D.
	Humble, Rosanna B.	Washington, Leonard

Source: *Flint Medical College, Department of Pharmacy, New Orleans University, Sarah Goodrich Hospital Nursing Training School and Department of Midwifery, Session 1914-1915* (New Orleans, LA: New Orleans University, 1915), 47-49.

TABLE 21. Geographical Distribution of New Orleans University College of Pharmacy Graduates after Graduation from 1903 to 1913

State	Number (%)
Alabama	2 (4)
Arkansas	1 (2)
Georgia	2 (4)
Louisiana	30 (59)
Mississippi	8 (16)
Oklahoma	2 (4)
Texas	5 (10)

Sources: New Orleans University, *Tan and Blue Annual Catalogue Edition, New Orleans University 1913-1914.* E.T. Harvey & Son: New Orleans, LA, 1914, accessed January 10, 2016, http://hdl.handle.net/2027/uiuo.ark:/13960/t7dr4fc96

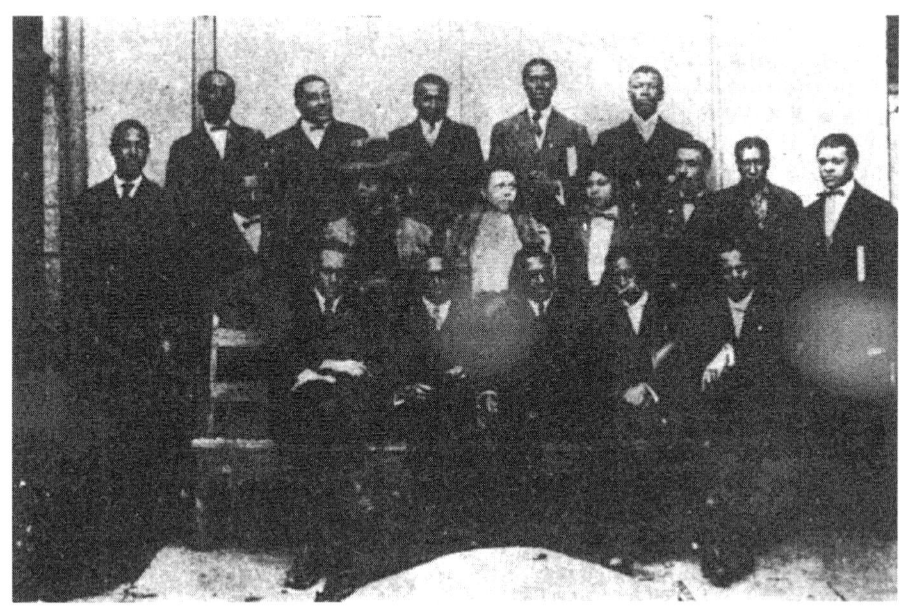

FIGURE 30. Pharmacy Class of 1907, New Orleans University College of Pharmacy.

(Source: *Annual Catalogue, New Orleans University, 1907-1908, 35th Session* [New Orleans, LA: Merchants Printing Co., Ltd, 1908], 47.)

In 1915, the New Orleans University College of Pharmacy closed.[318] That year all of the buildings of the Flint Medical College were placed under the use of the Sarah Goodridge Hospital, which continued to operate under the administration of the Methodist Episcopal Church. In 1916 a renovation was done on the facilities, which had fallen into disrepair.[319] In June 1930, New Orleans University and Straight College (formerly Straight University) merged and opened as Dillard University, as it is known today. The Sarah Goodridge Hospital and Nurse Training School was renamed Flint-Goodridge Hospital of Dillard University in 1932 and continued to be operated by Dillard University until 1983.[320]

6 Louisville National Medical College Pharmaceutical Department

John E. Clark

The Louisville National Medical College (LNMC) was incorporated in the state of Kentucky on April 24, 1888. The school was founded by three African American physicians: Dr. William Henry Fitzbutler, Dr. William A. Burney, and Dr. Rufus Conrad. LNMC started as one of the most promising medical schools in the South for African Americans. Initially, it was the only medical college in the U.S. that was managed entirely by African Americans. It began with a strong and prominent Board of Directors, which included the likes of Bishop Henry McNeal Turner,[321] Booker T. Washington,[322] Thomas William Haigler,[323] and many others.[324] It also had a highly qualified and motivated faculty (see **Figure 31**), a hospital for training and providing direct patient care, along with a dispensary and laboratory for the training of its students in the pharmaceutical and medical sciences. (See **Figure 32**.)

The Pharmaceutical Department opened with the start of the 1902–1903 session.[325] There were two academic sessions divided into 12-week terms for 24 weeks each year. Advertisements were published in several newspapers to recruit students and provide a brief description of the Department of Pharmacy and the length of the program. (See **Figure 33**.) The pharmacy program was later increased to three sessions, continuous for 28 weeks in 1903,[326] and again to 30 weeks in 1907.[327] The cost for tuition was $30.00 per session.[328]

Like other African American pharmacy programs, the admission policy and practices were very similar, if not the same, as the Medical College. Conditions for admission included: (1) Written documentation certifying good moral character (e.g., letters of reference); (2) Preliminary education, including at least a high school diploma; and (3) Satisfactorily passing examinations in the subjects of Algebra, Composition and Rhetoric, English literature, Latin, Geometry, History, Physics and Civics.[329] Although age, gender, or race were not included in their course announcements, the school had an open admission policy and admitted both males and females.

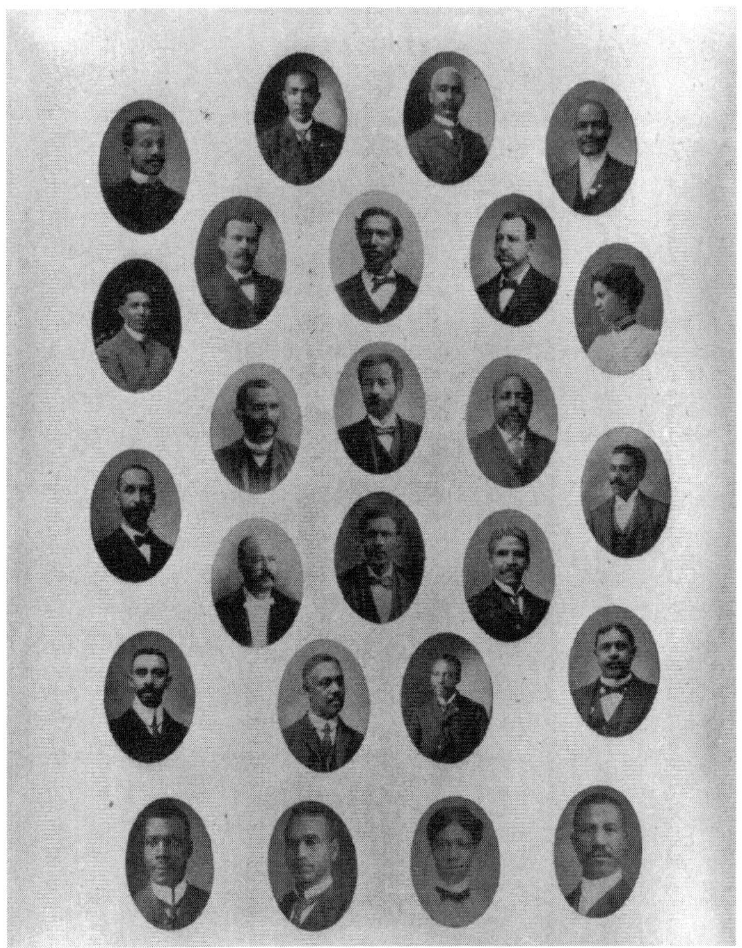

FIGURE 31. Founding Faculty, 1888-1889, Louisville National Medical College.

(Source: Louisville National Medical College, History Collection. *Louisville National Medical College records, 1888-1908.* [Louisville, KY: Kornhauser Health Sciences Library, University of Louisville].)

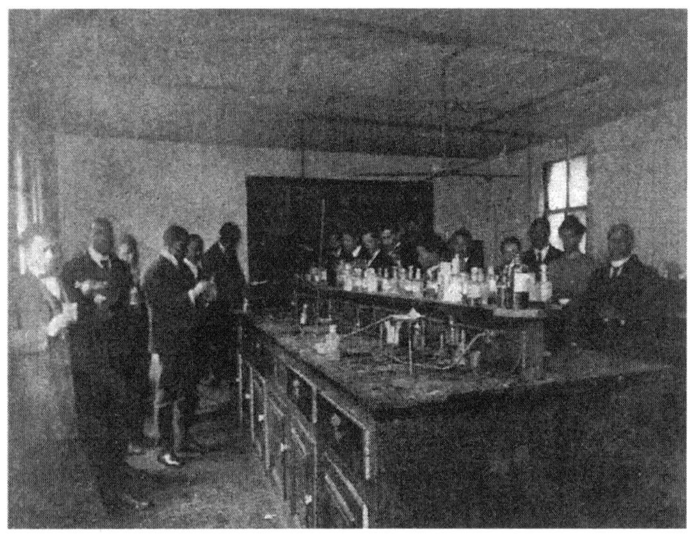

FIGURE 32. Medical and Pharmaceutical Laboratory, Louisville National Medical College, 1907.

(Source: Louisville National Medical College, History Collection, *Louisville National Medical College records, 1888-1908.* [Louisville, KY: Kornhauser Health Sciences Library, University of Louisville].)

STUDY MEDICINE AND PHARMACY AT THE

Louisville National Medical College

FIFTEENTH YEAR.

Recognized by all State Boards. All buildings are the property of the School, and have been entirely remodeled with fully equipped Laboratories and Hospital.

Nearly 100 Graduates in various parts of the country, every one of them enjoying a lucrative practice.

School of Medicine. Four years of six months each. Session continues throughout the year. Each session is divided into four terms of three months each. Attendance upon any two terms entitles student to credit for one year's attendance.

Terms: January, April, July and October. Examinations at end of each term. Students may enter at beginning of any term.

Department of Pharmacy. Two years, six months each session is divided into two terms of three months each.

For further informatiou and Catalogue address

W. A. BURNEY, M. D., Dean, Louisville, Ky.

Figure 33. Advertisement to Study Medicine and Pharmacy at Louisville National Medical College.

(Source: *The Freedman [Newspaper],* August 2, 1902, 5.)

The pharmacy course of study included:

- *First Year*: Pharmacy, *Materia Medica*, Botany, Chemistry, and Chemical Laboratory Work.
- *Second Year*: Pharmaceutical Laboratory Work, Qualitative Analysis, *Materia Medical,* Pharmacognosy, Toxicology, and Pharmacy.
- *Third Year*: Volumetric and gravimetric Analysis, Milk and Water Analysis, Microscopy, Hygiene, Urinalysis, Synthetic Chemistry, and Pharmacy.[330]

To graduate, the candidate: (1) Had to be at least 21 years of age, in good moral character; (2) Must have attended at least three sessions of pharmaceutical education and instructions; and (3) Satisfactorily pass examinations in all subject areas in the curriculum. Upon completion of the requirements, the candidate would be awarded the Pharmaceutical Chemist (Ph.C.) degree.[331] Those who had completed a medical or dental course of study at the LNMC or at some other reputable college, would also be allowed to complete the pharmacy course of study in two sessions.[332]

The Pharmacy Department maintained a well-stocked pharmaceutical laboratory, equipped with all the latest drugs and drug products conducive for the complete training of students in the preparation and dispensing of pharmaceuticals. Many of the drugs and drug products were donated by Sharpe & Dohme (today Merck & Co.). Lectures, recitations, and demonstrations were given four times a week during the first semester of the first year, and during the second semester of the second year. The Pharmacology and Therapeutics course was taught throughout the Junior year with lectures, recitations, and demonstrations. The first part of the course was devoted to general pharmacology. After the first month, individual drugs were presented, while discussing their therapeutic use, pharmacologic effects, mechanisms of actions, and adverse effects.

The "Preparation of Medicine" course was taught with a as series of lectures initially, followed by one-hour lectures once a week throughout the year. The course was taught in a manner that more directly benefited the medical students, although it was taught in the

Department of Pharmacy. The course included exercises in prescribing and prescription writing of the most prescribed drugs.

The second year was comprised of practical work in pharmacy, qualitative and quantitative analysis, and toxicology.[333]

The Department of Pharmacy faculty was made up of primarily the physicians from the Medical Department. The only two pharmacy trained faculty were Dr. Otto Oppelt, Ph.D., Ph.G., Professor of Pharmacy and Pharmaceutical Chemistry[334] and Dr. R. F. (Randolph F.) White, Phar.D. (Howard, 1897), Professor of Inorganic Chemistry and Instructor of Laboratory Chemistry.[335] In 1902, Dr. Oppelt was listed as the Dean of the LNMC Department of Pharmacy, succeeding Dr. W. A. Burney, M.D., who had been listed as Dean in many of the school's annual announcements and newspaper recruitment advertisements.[336] (See **Figure 33**.) He attended the University of Leipzig in Leipzig, Germany. He moved to New Albany, Indiana where he became a registered pharmacist and opened a drug store at 604 State Street.[337] Being very active and respected in the community, he would occasionally be called upon to serve as an expert witness in legal cases involving chemicals.[338] Around the same time when he joined the LNMC, he received national attention when he was issued a patent in 1903 for developing an improved process for producing natural gas at a lower cost than the standard production methods.[339] It seemed like a very promising business venture, but he was never able to capitalized financially on his discovery.[340]

The most recognized figure behind the LNMC was the founder and Dean, Dr. William Henry Fitzbutler. Dr. Fitzbutler was born in Ontario, Canada in 1842. In 1871, he was the first African American student to enroll in the Detroit Medical College. He transferred to the University of Michigan and became the first African American to graduate from the College of Medicine in 1872.[341] The same year, he moved to Louisville, Kentucky where he was the first African American physician in the city at the time. Immediately, he became heavily involved in civil rights, social and political issues in the community. He was a strong and devoted advocate of medical education for African Americans, which led him and his partners to establish the Louisville National Medical College. The school was almost completely financed with their own funds, including the purchase of its buildings and an auxiliary hospital. His wife, Sarah

McCurdy Fitzbutler and three of their children, John Henry, Marie, and Prima Fitzbutler, all graduated as physicians from the LNMC.[342]

Dr. Henry Fitzbutler, as he was called, was a business man, politician, and publisher of his own newspaper, *The Ohio Falls Express*.[343] He also delved heavily into the local and state politics during a time of declining racial status and relations for African Americans in the South. He aspired to be a political leader in the Republican Party and was often not in good favor with blacks and whites for his stance on racial and social injustice. Some black leaders considered him among the "black militant leaders"[344] and bitterly opposed him personally in a number of local and state leadership battles, including elections to the city school board,[345] delegate to state and national Republican conventions,[346] and chair and leadership roles in various committees within the political party.[347] One black church leader caused his arrest by filing criminal libel charges against him claiming he published false and damaging reports about his character in his newspaper.[348] Because of his strong and outspoken personality, he was also frequently challenged with threats and attempts of expulsion from various local and state political committees. An attempt was once made to have him expelled from the Republican party for voting against a Republican congressional nominee.[349]

Some of the challenges also filtered into his role as Dean of LNMC and as a healthcare provider. He was called upon in April 1894 to testify and defend the operations of the medical school in front of the Kentucky State Board of Health regarding allegations that one of the female graduates ("school mistress") had received a diploma without attending classes. He defended himself and four other such cases so well that the Board approved the issuance of the diplomas to the graduates and recognized LNMC as following the same minimum standards as white schools of medicine.[350]

He was arrested and accused of murder of a young white female patient that was brought to him for an abortion by her boyfriend and who died after developing septicemia following a surgical procedure allegedly performed by Dr. Fitrzbutler.[351] The case was later dismissed for lack of sufficient evidence.[352]

To improve the teaching and to acquire knowledge of the most efficient techniques and modern medical tools, Dr. Fitzbutler toured and visited hospitals in New York, London, and other English cities of the UK. While traveling in England, Dr. Fitzbutler developed very severe bronchitis. Upon returning home, he did not recover and died from his illness on December 28, 1901.[353] His death led to several lawsuits over his assets, involving disputes between the state,[354] his family,[355] and between the family and one of his founding partners.[356]

Shortly thereafter, the standards at the school started to decline, but not just because of Dr. Fitzbutler's death. LNMC faced mounting pressure from requirements associated with medical education reform. To meet these higher standards, LNMC added faculty, lengthened the curriculum, strengthened the graduation and admission requirements, increased the laboratory and clinical experience, and added an auxiliary hospital.

LNMC also entered an affiliation with State University Medical Department in 1903 and became Louisville National Medical College, Department of Medicine and Pharmacy of State University. The Department of Pharmacy faculty included:

- Otto Oppelt, Ph.D., Ph.G., *Professor of Pharmacy and Pharmaceutical Chemistry*
- N.S. Fuller, M.D., *Professor of Materia Medica*
- Clarkson W. Houser, M.D., *Professor of Chemistry*
- Prima Fitzbutler, M.D., *Professor of Botany.*[357]

Still, the administration found it increasingly difficult to obtain sufficient funding to offset escalating costs associated with the rising standard of education at the college. The school had no steady stream of income beyond that of tuition. There was no financial support from the state or federal government, nor support from the religious organizations. No student loans were available. Many of the medical services at the auxiliary hospital were free to qualified patients and generated no steady revenue. The practicing physicians and surgeons had to cover their own expense for operating in the hospital.

After the school was reviewed for accreditation, it was found that LNMC had an unsatisfactory passing rate by graduates on the state medical licensing examinations.[358] Ultimately, this poor graduate performance combined with the mounting financial pressures led to the school's closing in 1912. The Pharmacy Department was closely linked to the Medical Department and soon closed around the same time.

The total number of students who enrolled and the total number of graduates in the LNMC Department of Pharmacy is unknown. Like other similar pharmacy programs, the numbers were very small. Between 1902 and 1908, LNMC graduated two students from the Department of Pharmacy with the Ph.C. degree:

1. Jessie Merchant (1904)
2. E. D. (Edward D.) Morrison (1906)

Miss M. E. (Mary E.) Jarman is listed as the only pharmacy student in the 1906-1907 class, but she does not appear in the list of graduates in the 1908 or 1909 class.[359] It is not clear whether Jesse Merchant and Edward D. Morrison were able to establish a pharmacy practice, i.e., become registered pharmacists. Edward D. Morrison is listed in the 1907 *U.S. City Directories* database as a porter employed at the Citizens' National Hospital in Louisville, KY, the auxiliary teaching hospital for the LNMC Departments of Medicine.[360] Jessie Merchant had been extremely active in community and civic activities throughout his life. He served as civilian post-master for the 10th U.S. Volunteer Infantry at Lexington, KY and Macon, GA during the Spanish-American War. He was a poet and orator and was credited with composing the lyrics to the song, *Back to My Old Kentucky Home* in 1906. In 1909, Jessie Merchant moved to Chicago after graduation. He used his Pharmaceutical Chemist (Ph.C.) degree to obtain work as a chemist in the alcohol tax unit laboratory of the Internal Revenue Service in Chicago. He was with the government laboratory for 41 years, spending 10 years with the Department of Agriculture in the U.S. Food Laboratory section before joining the alcohol testing laboratory during prohibition in the early 1920s. Jesse Merchant's laboratory job during prohibition was to test samples of whisky, beer, and other forms of liquor to determine whether they contained a sufficient concentration of alcohol to support the government's cases against "bootleggers." Because of the sensitivity of his work and the potential for corruption and retaliation, his name and contact information were kept confidential by the Treasury Department for a long time, along with undercover agents, inspectors, and investigators.

In March 1929, Senator R. F. Wagner (D, N.Y.) sponsored a resolution calling upon the Treasury Department and the Civil Service Commission to release the names to the public of all personnel involved with prohibition, and to explain the secrecy surrounding the persons on the list.[361]

It is very likely that there were more pharmacy graduates from LNMC than what are reported here. The records that would help confirm the actual numbers, as well as the more detailed information about the pharmacy program, appears to have been lost with the closing of the school.

7 Frelinghuysen University School of Pharmacy

John E. Clark, Raisah Salhab

The Frelinghuysen University was a school formed in the Washington, District of Columbia (D. C.) to meet the educational needs of working-class African Americans who wanted to continue their education and maintain their full-time employment. Classes were held at night and at times outside the normal business hours. Since the school did not start with a campus or a permanent building, classes were held in private homes and businesses until 1921 when a new building was constructed at 601 M Street N.W.[362]

The school evolved from a branch of the Bible Educational Association and the Interdenominational Bible College in 1906 and was later referred as the Interdenominational University. Dr. Jesse and Rosetta C. Lawson are credited as the founders of the school. Dr. Lawson was personal friends with John Mercer Langston and Booker T. Washington, and many other acquaintances in the D.C. area. He was also highly esteemed by Senator Frederick Theodore Frelinghuysen, Sr. On February 22, 1917, the Board of Directors of the Interdenominational University voted to officially change the name of the school to the Frelinghuysen University in honor of the U.S. senator from New Jersey who had been an active supporter of civil rights while serving in the Senate.

The university was made up of a group of schools which included an Academy, a Business High School, School of Liberal Arts, School of Applied Sciences, School of Theology, School of Law, School of Chiropractic, School of Sociology, School of Embalming and Sanitary Science, and a School of Pharmacy.

The School of Pharmacy started in 1917. The classes were held on Tuesday, Thursday, Friday and Saturday evenings each week, from 7 p.m. to 11 p.m. Admission was open to both men and women, with no restrictions because of race or religion. Applicants had to be at least 17 years of age; have completed eight years of study in secondary school; at least one year of Latin; and be morally fit. Applicants who had spent time in a drugstore received credit for their practice experience.

The annual sessions of the School of Pharmacy were 32 weeks, starting in the Fall (October) and ending in the Spring. The tuition was $60.00 per scholastic year, plus other fees for laboratory, books, and graduation. After three years of course work and meeting all requirements, students were to be awarded the degree of Doctor of Pharmacy (Phar.D.).

A detail description of the curriculum is unclear. The curriculum included courses in Chemistry, Toxicology, Botany, Materia Medica, Therapeutics, Pharmacy, Pharmacology, Physiology, and Bacteriology. The classes were small and limited by classroom and laboratory space. The courses at the beginning of the 1920 session were taught primarily by four pharmacy faculty members with strong connections to the Howard University Pharmaceutical College.[363] (See **Table 22.**)

TABLE 22. Frelinghuysen University School of Pharmacy Faculty: 1920–1921

Name	Rank	Course
William H. Jackson, Phar.D.	Dean, Professor	Mercantile Pharmacy
Herbert C. Scurlock, A.M., M.D.	Professor	Chemistry
Joseph D. Smith, Phar.D.	Professor	Materia Media, Therapeutics and Toxicology
Edward F. Harris, Phar.D.	Professor	Pharmacy Practice (Caspari) and Botany

Source: *Courses of Study in the Frelinghuysen University of Washington, D.C., 1920-1921.*(Washington, DC: The Frelinghuysen University, 1920)

Dr. William H. Jackson, Dean and Professor of the School of Pharmacy, was a 1904 (Phar.D.) graduate of Howard University. He came to the attention of the Frelinghuysen School of Pharmacy from the firm of Jackson & Whipps, a retail pharmacy center located at Seventh and T Streets Northwest, in which he was a partner with fellow colleague, William W. Whipps, Phar.D. (Howard, 1903). Dr. Jackson taught courses from the business aspects of pharmacy practice. His pharmacy was also listed in the early course catalogue as a place where students could acquire valuable practice experience in understanding the business of operating a pharmacy. He was active locally in the D.C. Druggists' Association and the National Medical Association (NMA). He served as Chair of the Executive Committee of the D.C. Druggists' Association and was elected Chairman of the Pharmaceutical Section of the NMA in 1919.[364]

Dr. Herbert C. Scurlock was a longtime faculty member of the Howard University College of Pharmacy. He graduated in the 1900 class of the Howard University College of Medicine and served as Professor of Chemistry from 1898-1940.[365] He taught Chemistry at Howard during the day and at Frelinghuysen University at night.

Dr. Edward F. Harris (Phar.D.) was Professor of Pharmacy Practice and taught courses in Pharmacy and Botany. He was a local activist, businessman, former military officer (Army 2nd Lieutenant), and the Secretary of the D.C. Druggists' Association. In April 1919, he led the efforts in campaigning and filing the petition with the D.C. Supreme Court for Walter C. Simmons, Phar.D. (Howard, 1909), President of the D.C. Druggists' Association, who had been unanimously selected as a candidate for the Washington Board of Education.[366] He also served as the editor of the *Journal of the National Medical Association* Pharmaceutical Section. Dr. Harris published several of the papers and speeches presented by pharmacists at NMA Annual meetings in the Pharmaceutical Section of the Journal.[367]

Dr. Joseph D. Smith (Phar.D.) was the fourth member that made up the pharmacy faculty. He was a highly regarded pharmacists who taught the courses in Materia Medica, Therapeutics, and Toxicology.

On November 5, 1927, President and Founder of Frelinghuysen University, Dr. Jesse Lawson dies.[368]In 1929, Dr. Anna J. Cooper, noted educator, author, and sociologist, was elected President of Frelinghuysen University but was not inducted until June 1930. She started with "bewildering" debt, no endowments, no student scholarships, or financial appropriations other than tuition. After much work to raise money and to re-distribute the little available financial resources for the basic operations of the school, her efforts were not enough to maintain the mortgage on some of the buildings and the income from student enrollment and tuition. The debt increased, the banks would not extend credit, foreclosures occurred on some properties, and no government assistance was provided despite her well-known political contacts. She moved the classes into her own home temporarily at 201 T Street NW. By the mid-1930s, the Washington Board of Education, being the only organization to recognize a school as a University, refused to approve degree offerings and to accredit the school's academic programs. Despite an intense court battle to appeal the decision, the Frelinghuysen University lost its charter in 1937 and in the 1940s, re-open as the (non-degree) Frelinghuysen Group of Schools for Colored Working People. The school was later dissolved in the 1950s.[369]

It is unclear when the decision was made to discontinue the School of Pharmacy. The pharmacy program was last mentioned in reports about the school in 1926. While several students were listed by class years in the 1920-1921 Course Study,[370] it is also unclear how many students were awarded the Phar.D. degree from the Frelinghuysen University or became registered pharmacists. (See **Table 23**)

TABLE 23. Students of the Frelinghuysen University School of Pharmacy: 1920–1924

CLASS	NAME	
1921	Jackson, Bertie Beard	Turner, Jerry
	Jordan, James	Ussery, Harry H.
	Smith, Ollie F.	Ussery, Margaret E.
1922	Johnson, Leroy E.	
	Peebles, Frank R.	
1923	Alexander, Theodore	Ryce, Oscar Andrew
	Baker, John H.	Twine, Charles A.
	Brown, Ernest D.	Wines, Harold
	Challoner, Robert L.	Williams, Wymoning
	Early, James Harvey	West, William
	Palms, Thomas Phillip	
1924	Ward, Jerry W.	

Source: *Courses of Study in the Frelinghuysen University of Washington, D.C., 1920-1921.*(Washington, DC: The Frelinghuysen University, 1920); "Many Given Degrees, Frelinghuysen University Graduates Receive Honors," *Evening Star,* June 7, 1924, 4.

Discussion and Summary

There were nine pharmacy schools established for training African Americans during the period from 1868–1937. Seven of the schools have since closed, but not before issuing over 700 pharmacy diplomas to its graduates. In the first ten years of their existence, all the schools graduated small numbers of students ranging from 1 to 12 graduates per year. Over time, the number of graduates gradually increased, as was seen with Meharry Pharmaceutical College in 1922 when 43 pharmacy students were issued diplomas. At the time, this was the largest graduation class ever of African American pharmacy students in the country. After graduation, the graduates became pharmacists in at least 33 states and two foreign countries.[371]

Most all the early African American pharmacists and pharmacy schools evolved around African American physicians and their medical school programs, as well as their professional association. The African American physicians who owned drug stores were also some of the first to train African American pharmacy apprentices, employ African American pharmacy graduates, and to provide a site for many to acquire the experience needed to take the pharmacy licensure examination to become a pharmacist.[372] Some of the most well-known physicians included: James McCune Smith, M.D.,[373] Peter William Ray, M.D.,[374] Lincoln Laconia (L.L.) Burwell, M.D.,[375] George Samuel Pryce, M.D.,[376] Henry Rutherford Butler, M.D., and many more who not only opened very successful drugstores along with their medical practice (see **Figure 34**), but were also registered pharmacists.[377]

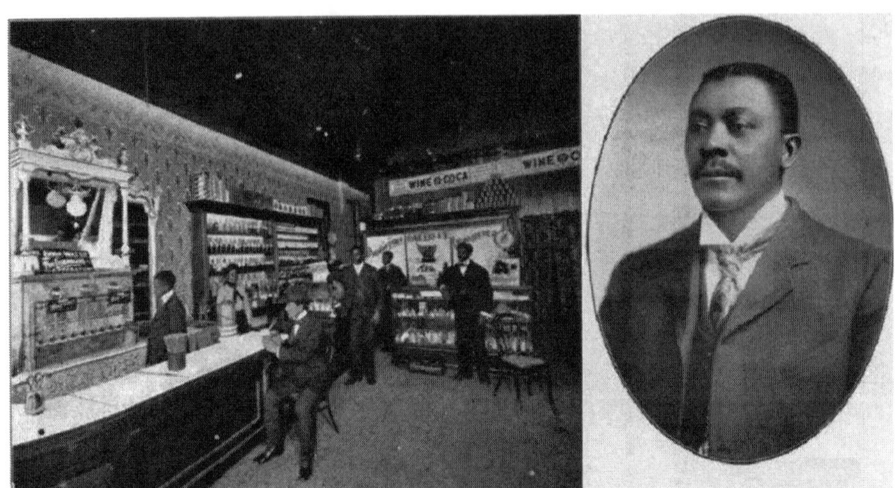

FIGURE 34. Dr. L. L. Burwell and His Pharmacy in Selma, AL, 1907.

(Source: Robinson, Wilhelmena S. *International Library of Negro Life and History – The History of the Negro in Medicine*. [New York, NY: Publishers Company, Inc., 1969], 68.)

From the late 1890s to early 1900s, there was very little participation and inclusion of African American pharmacists as members in local, state, and pharmacy associations, largely because the practice of segregation was embraced complicitly by many of the organizations. The National Medical Association (NMA) was one of the only professional association that openly welcomed and encouraged the participation of African American pharmacists as members. When the NMA was formed in 1895, it was originally founded as the National Association of Colored Physicians, Dentists, and Pharmacists, then referred to the National Medical, Dental, and Pharmaceutical Association, and later the name was changed to the National Medical Association.

While there is no evidence that the American Pharmaceutical Association (APhA), or other professional pharmacy associations, systematically excluded African American pharmacists, there is also no evidence that they presented resolutions to break down the barriers for their participation. Some members openly opposed the membership of African American pharmacists. In 1892, members of the Alabama

Pharmaceutical Association (an APhA state affiliate) opposed the membership of John Darius Crum, an African American pharmacist from Selma, who joined the APhA without mention of his race in the membership application process.[378] The concerned Alabama members became so outraged by the incident that they filed a complaint with their Executive Committee for the expulsion of Mr. Albert E. Brown, a member who had endorsed Mr. Crum for membership in the APhA. The pharmacists registering the complaint felt Mr. Brown had offended the State of Alabama and its members of the Association, and strongly criticized his action for endorsing Mr. Crum's application. The Executive Committee decided that Mr. Brown had committed no offense against the state association. The Committee further explained that this was a membership matter for the national organization (APhA) and for the APhA to decide if charges should be brought against Mr. Brown. The APhA accepted John Darius Crum's membership as his name is listed among Active Members in a report given at the APhA 43rd Annual Meeting in 1895.[379] It is not certain when the APhA started granting membership to African American pharmacists. Mr. Crum is likely among the first African American pharmacists to join the APhA, especially from the South.

Attending Association sponsored meetings, conferences, entertainment, and social events may have also offered challenges for African American pharmacists. From the 1890s to the 1960s, many places in the South where APhA annual meetings were held embraced practices of segregation ("Jim Crow"), which restricted African American pharmacists who might have wanted to attend the meetings from participating in conference hotels, restaurants, and other public places.

Polk Miller was a pharmacist, an APhA member, and an entertainer who was scheduled several times to perform for members at APhA meetings.[380] He and his sons own the successful Polk Miller Drug and Chemical Company in Richmond, Virginia.[381] He was a former soldier who fought for the Confederacy, grew up on a Virginia plantation, and glorified and presented black music in the "Negro dialect."[382] His performances were openly nostalgic for the days of slavery, and his music was very entertaining and popular to many members and the public. Although he had a very rare and unique band and was one of the first popular white entertainers in America to perform in front of audiences with black band members, none of his performances called for African American equality, integration, or unity among all pharmacists, but instead frequently affirmed and perpetuated negative stereotypes of African Americans and of the slaves he had own on his plantation.[383]

In the NMA, African American pharmacists could freely attend and present as speakers at national conventions, serve as delegates in the NMA House of Delegates, serve on committees, the executive board, and publish articles in their professional journal (JNMA), which they did quite actively.[384] To create a collegial place for African American pharmacists, the NMA also formed several affiliate state and regional chapters. Some of the chapters still exist today. (See **Table 24**.) The strong relationship between African American physicians and pharmacists remained for decades, but began to change somewhat from the 1920s to the 1940s with low participation and modest growth in the pharmacists' membership. In 1947, under the leadership of Dr. Chauncey Cooper, African American pharmacists formed the National Pharmaceutical Association (NPhA), which became the first professional pharmacy association to foster collaboration, advocacy, education, and leadership for black pharmacists and black patients. The second national pharmacy association advocating for black pharmacists and patients was started when the Association of Black Hospital Pharmacists was formed in 1979.

TABLE 24. Medical, Dental, and Pharmaceutical Associations in the United States: 1914–1915

- Alabama Medical, Dental, and Pharmaceutical Association
- Arkansas Medical, Dental, and Pharmaceutical Association
- Florida Medical, Dental, and Pharmaceutical Association
- Tri-County Medical, Dental, and Pharmaceutical Association of Florida
- Indiana Association of Physicians, Dentists, and Pharmacists
- Kentucky Medical, Dental, and Pharmaceutical Association
- Louisiana Medical, Dental, and Pharmaceutical Association
- Maryland Medical, Dental, and Pharmaceutical Association
- Massachusetts Medical, Dental, and Pharmaceutical Association
- Mississippi Medical, Dental, and Pharmaceutical Association
- North Carolina Medical, Dental, and Pharmaceutical Association
- Palmetto Medical, Dental, and Pharmaceutical Association
- Lone State Medical, Dental, and Pharmaceutical Association
- Atlanta Association of Negro Physicians, Dentists, and Pharmacists
- Physicians, Dentists, and Pharmacists Club of Chicago
- Philadelphia Academy of Medicine and the Allied Sciences
- Bluff City Medical, Dental, and Pharmaceutical Society of Memphis Tennessee
- Dallas Negro Medical, Dental, and Pharmaceutical Association

Source: Work, Monroe Nathan. *Negro Year Book: An Annual Encyclopedia of the Negro, 1914-1915*. (Tuskegee, Ala.: Negro Year Book Publication, 1914.)

Although there are several factors that can be attributable to the evolution, slow rise, and integration of African American pharmacists, one of the most important factors was the creation of the African American pharmacy schools.[385] While there were questions raised about the education, training, and competence of the pharmacy graduates, the schools had about as much in common between them as they did differences with the predominately white schools in the same state.[386] In a very general and limited comparison, admission and graduation requirements, course content and length of the curriculum were similar (varied slightly by 1-2 weeks), as well as the size of graduating classes and faculty. The tuition cost and fees were slightly lower at the African American pharmacy schools than the predominately white schools in the same state. (See **Table 25**.) All the schools started as a 2-year program and seem to have increased their curriculum to a 3-year program by the second or third class. Meharry Pharmaceutical College was the only African American school that was a member of the American Conference of Pharmaceutical Faculties (ACPF).[387] The curriculum of the other African American schools closely resembled that of Meharry and thus that of some of the predominately white pharmacy schools that were members of the ACPF at the time.

In 1895, it was not uncommon for some of the pharmacy schools to not require drug store experience as a requirement for graduation. Depending on the pharmacy degree being conferred, some Schools of Pharmacy, such as the University of Wisconsin[388] and the University of Minnesota,[389] did not require drugstore experience to graduate. Vanderbilt University Department of Pharmacy, located in the same state as Meharry and University of West Tennessee, also did not require students to have drugstore experience to graduate, if the Ph.C. degree was to be awarded.[390]

The Ph.C. degree was one of several common degrees issued by Departments and Colleges of Pharmacy early on. Depending on the school, the pharmacy degrees could include the Ph.C. (2 year), Ph.G. (2 year), Phar.D. (2-4 year), or the B.S. (4 year). Most Ph.C. graduates had the options of teaching, working in scientific laboratories, or state government departments without being licensed. However, if they chose pharmacy practice, hours of drug store experience were required to take the state licensing examination, much of which could be acquired after graduation.[391]

TABLE 25. Early African American Pharmacy Schools Comparison: 1890–1912

Characteristics	Meharry Pharmaceutical Department[1]	University of West Tennessee[2] Pharmaceutical Department	Vanderbilt University Department of Pharmacy[3]
Admission Requirements	Good moral character, English; pre-examination; Latin; women & blacks accepted	18 years old; good moral character; pre-examination, Latin, English; women accepted	16 years old, good English education, moral character; women accepted; blacks not accepted
Cost per Session			
Tuition	$30	$40 (+ labs)	$50
Graduating fee	$10	$10	$5
Chem, Pharm lab	$8	—	$35
Matriculation	—	—	$10
Board & Lodging	$10/mo.	$10/mo.	$13-18/mo.
Books	—	—	$15
Length of term	20 weeks	24 weeks	32 weeks
Number of terms	3	3	2
Graduation Requirements	• 21 yrs. of age • Pass examination • Complete 3 sessions + 4 yrs. practice experience, inclusive	• 21 yrs. of age • Pass examination • Completed 3 sessions	• No experience required (Ph.C.), 3 yrs… course (Ph.M.); 4 yrs. required (Ph.G.)
Training Opportunities	Pharmacy practice during sessions	Some dispensary opportunities	Campus pharmacy lab; Drug store
Degree Conferred	Ph.C.	Ph.C.	Ph.C., Ph.G., Ph.M.
M.D.	3	2	3
PhC, Phar.D.,	4	2	2
Ph.G. Ph.D., MS			2
Faculty (No. tot.)	7	4	7
# of Students grad, approx. avg./yr	6	5	4

TABLE 25. Early African American Pharmacy Schools Comparison: 1890–1912 (Continued)

Characteristics	Shaw Leonard School of Pharmacy[4]	University of North Carolina Department of Pharmacy[5]	New Orleans University College of Pharmacy[6]
Admission Requirements	Good English education; proficiency in Latin; women accepted	Good English; blacks not accepted	18 years old; good moral character; high school or college; women accepted;
Cost per Session			
Tuition	$25	$30	$40
Graduating fee	$10	—	$10
Chem, Pharm lab	—	$1.25-5	$10
Matriculation	$5	—	$5
Board & Lodging	$8.50/mo.	$8-$13/mo.	$12-$15/mo.
Books	$10	—	$18
Length of term	32 weeks	36 weeks	30 weeks
Number of terms	3	2	3
Graduation Requirements	• 21 yrs. of age • Pass examination • Complete 3 sessions	• No experience required	• 21 yrs. of age • Pass examination • Complete 3 sessions
Training Opportunities	Pharmacy Lab. attached to Dispensary on campus	Pharmacy lab	Pharmacy dispensing lab. during sessions, 150 hrs.
Degree Conferred	Ph.C.	Ph.G.	Ph.G.
M.D.		1	6
PhC, Phar.D.,	3	1	2
Ph.G. Ph.D., MS	1	5	
Faculty (No. tot.)	4	7	8
# of Students grad, approx. avg./yr	5	17	5

TABLE 25. Early African American Pharmacy Schools Comparison: 1890–1912 (Continued)

Characteristics	Tulane University Department of Pharmacy[7]	Louisville National Medical College[8,9] Pharmaceutical Department	Louisville College of Pharmacy[9]
Admission Requirements	21 yrs old, moral character; reputable women, no black admitted	Unclear; same as the medical college, pre-examination, high school or other	Good English education;
Cost per Session			
Tuition	$75-$80/yr.	$30	$60-$85/yr.
Graduating fee	$20	$10	$10
Chem, Pharm lab	$15	—	—
Matriculation	$5	—	—
Board & Lodging	$18-22/mo.	—	—
Books	—	—	—
Length of term	—	30 weeks	24 weeks
Number of terms	2	3	2
Graduation Requirements	• 21 yrs. of age; • Two yrs. course experience	• Pass an examination; complete 3 sessions	• 21 yrs. of age • Four yrs. of experience
Training Opportunities	Pharmacy and chemical lab on campus	Pharmacy dispensary present	—
Degree Conferred	Ph.G.	Ph.G.	Ph.G.
M.D.	—	1	—
PhC, Phar.D.,	—	4	—
Ph.G. Ph.D., MS	—	—	—
Faculty (No. tot.)	—	5	—
# of Students grad, approx. avg./yr	10	Uncertain	—

TABLE 25. Early African American Pharmacy Schools Comparison: 1890–1912 (Concluded)

Source: [1]Meharry Medical College, *"1910 Meharry Medical College Catalogue," Meharry Medical College Archives*, accessed January 22, 2016, http://diglib.mmc.edu/omeka/items/show/103; [2]University of West Tennessee, *"Catalogue for the Session of 1909-1910. Announcement for the Session of 1910-1911."* (Memphis, TN: University of West Tennessee, 1910); [3]*Register of Vanderbilt University for 1893-94, Announcement for 1894-95* (Nashville, TN: Vanderbilt University, 1894); [4]Leonard Medical School, *"Annual Catalog of the Officers and Students of Leonard School of Pharmacy, The Pharmaceutical Department of Shaw University. For the Academic Year ending May Thirty-first, Nineteen Hundred and Nine."* (Raleigh, NC: Leonard Medical School, 1909); [5]*The University of North Carolina Catalogue, 1897-98,* (Chapel Hill, NC: University of North Carolina, 1898); [6]New Orleans University, *"New Orleans University, 1912-1913,* (New Orleans, LA: ET Harvey & Sons, 1913);[7]*Tulane University of Louisiana, Medical Department 1898-1899,* (New Orleans, LA: Tulane University, 1899); [9]*"Our Pharmaceutical Colleges," Drug Circular Chemical Gazette, 41 (1897): 80-82.*

Most of the African American schools combined the hands-on laboratory practice experience in the preparation of prescription medicines with the classroom lectures. The hours required for graduation was not always clearly specified. Meharry started out requiring four years of practice experience in compounding and dispensing of medicines in a regular established pharmacy to receive the Graduate in Pharmacy degree (Ph.G.). The experience was inclusive of the practical experience in the classroom and laboratory. Being a two-year program at the time, approximately 80 hours (2 hours per day for 8 weeks) of compounding and dispensing experience was required in the second year of the program and the remainder of the experience was acquired after graduation.[392] In 1896, Meharry began awarding the Pharmaceutical Chemist (Ph.C.) degree. At the same time, the four years of practice experiences was no longer being listed in the catalogues as a requirement for receiving the Ph.C. degree. One year later, the length of the curriculum increased to three sessions. The pharmacy practice experience required in the curriculum also increased, primarily in the third year, and remained the same throughout the existence of the program.

The University of West Tennessee College of Pharmacy required laboratory work in the curriculum, but did not define the requirements for practice experience in processing prescriptions or the number of hours required in a drugstore.[393] Similarly, the New Orleans University College of Pharmacy and Louisville National Medical College Department of Pharmacy also included a large amount of pharmacy and laboratory work in all three years of their program, with most of the practice experience being acquired in their pharmaceutical or dispensing laboratory under the supervision of the faculty.[394] At the New Orleans University College of Pharmacy, a total of 100 hours of Pharmacy Practice experience was required in the first year, 90 hours in the second year, and 150 hours in the third year, but did not specify drugstore experience.[395]

Shaw Leonard School of Pharmacy advertised its program as having an advantage over other African American pharmacy schools around the same issue. In several of their catalogues, there were statements that students could acquire all the pharmacy practice experience in their pharmaceutical laboratory and the Leonard Dispensary, which suggested that they did not have to go outside of the school to do so.[396] Whether or not this influenced most students passing their licensure examination is uncertain. The New Orleans University College of Pharmacy did not seem to find drugstore experience to be an issue. In a section in the *Annual Catalogue of New Orleans University, 1907-1908,* it was stated ". . . . that our students of even the first and second years have been able, with no other instruction than that gotten here, to successfully pass the rigid examination of the State Boards."[397]

Four of the defunct African American pharmacy schools were directly affected by the recommendations in the 1910 Flexner Report. While the Report may have had good intentions, and the support of the AMA and the ACPF (today the AACP, American Association of Colleges of Pharmacy) as well,[398] like the African American medical schools, it had significant implications for African American pharmacy programs. Because the African American pharmacy programs were all departments within the medical schools, they became casualties of the racial biases that permeated the efforts to bring about reforms in medical education in the medical schools.[399] Not only did the recommendations to close the black medical schools lead to a reduction in African American physicians, it also reduced the number of African American pharmacists, the number of pharmacy-owned drugstores, and perpetuated discriminatory pharmaceutical (health) services in their communities.

It has been projected that the number of African Americans graduating from pharmacy schools in the U.S. fell to less than 20 students per year after the closing of the African American pharmacy programs.[400] With fewer students graduating and entering the profession, the number of African American-owned drugstores that would have been available to provide friendly access to pharmaceutical services also declined in some states.[401] In the 1920s, African Americans were reported to have owned 5 percent of the drugstores in the state of North Carolina. By the 1950s, that number had drastically declined and many of the stores closed.[402]

Access to basic health services became limited, especially in those white-owned drugstores where there were lunch counters and soda fountains. Because of such restrictions, the drugstores became a focal of point of protest throughout the South and in some other areas of the country during the Civil Rights Movement in the 1960s.[403]

The reduction in the number of African American owned drugstores may have also had an impact on other services besides the access to medicines. Some African American pharmacists served as primary care providers in underserved communities and was often referred to as “doctor” although they were pharmacists.[404] Their drugstores were often important centers of economic and social development. Some drugstore owners, for example, provided meeting rooms that may have been attached to the same building for African Americans to gather, as well as recreational facilities such as gymnasiums, barber services, libraries, and shops that may otherwise not have been available in the community to African Americans.[405]

Once the seven schools were closed, the only pharmacy schools for African Americans that remained opened were Howard University Pharmaceutical College and Xavier University of Louisiana College of Pharmacy. In a 1947 American Council of Education Pharmaceutical Survey, there were 20 out of 65 pharmacy schools that did not admit African American students.[406] They were all located in segregated areas of the South and in the same states where the African American pharmacy schools were forced to close. Findings and recommendations in the report raised questions about the impact of the closing of the pharmacy schools on the African American community. Three of the findings indicated:

1. *That the total number of existing drugstores is inadequate to render adequate health service to Negroes.*
2. *That each of the Southern states needs a 100 percent increase in the number of existing stores.*
3. *That there should be an increase of at least 10 to 15 percent in store ownership (by African Americans) within the next five-year period.*[407]

The author of the survey admits that the data may be limited but believes that the findings and recommendations are justifiable. After the report, two additional pharmacy schools at HBCUs were opened, which included Texas Southern University (then Texas State University for Negroes) School of Pharmacy (1948) and Florida A&M University College of Pharmacy (1951). Other HBCU pharmacy programs which were started years later included Hampton University School of Pharmacy (1997), Chicago State University (1998), and University of Maryland Eastern Shores (2010).

Although the six defunct African American pharmacy schools examined did not survive the change that was taking place in medicine and pharmacy at the time, these institutions made significant contributions to their communities and to the profession, as well as pave the way for the diversity and inclusion of African Americans that continues today.

Reflection

I graduated from the then FAMU (Florida A&M University) School of Pharmacy in 1961. After my first two years struggling as a registered African American pharmacist in Florida and Alabama, I had determined that retail pharmacy was not my bag. It was too "commercial", isolating and unfulfilling for me, particularly since at the time we could only work in Black-owned pharmacies in the South and pharmacists were not properly equipped to perform clinical services, especially in the retail environment. This meant low salaries and, in my case, even so, I had to be shared by two Black-owned pharmacies 40 miles apart with no reimbursement for travel expense (gas, etc.), owned by Simon Barnes in Delray Beach and James T. Houston, Jr., in Belle Glade, FL.

When I moved out to Birmingham, AL, in 1962 to work with a fellow FAMU pharmacist alumnus, Otis Williams, it was with a Walgreens Agency Drug Store owned by Black self-made millionaire, A.G. Gaston. Gaston owned the Booker T. Washington Insurance Co., a business college all housed in the AG Gaston Building, as well as a bank and real estate business housed nearby. This move gave me no increase in salary – only a better working environment. I was then recruited by a Xavier University pharmacy graduate, Eddie Clemons, who owned a small independent retail pharmacy in Mobile, AL. After those experiences, I was determined to move from retail pharmacy as a career to something more suitable to my abilities, interests and potential earnings. I, therefore, decided to go to graduate school to study industrial pharmacy.

When I enrolled in graduate studies in the College of Pharmacy at the University of Florida (UF) in August 1963, unknowing to me at the time, I became the first African American to enroll in the college at either the graduate or undergraduate level in the University's history. During the following two years each, not a single African American enrolled in the undergraduate pharmacy program there. I enrolled as an Industrial Pharmacy major with two minors. My first minor was pharmaceutical chemistry, and my second and extremely and surprisingly valuable minor was industrial and systems engineering, which proved to be one of the most beneficial decisions I made in my lifetime. It was against this background which provided me the personal background in industrial pharmacy and, subsequently, pharmacy practice, research, management and education locally, nationally and, eventually, internationally, to provide training materials prepared for and distributed by the U.S. Agency for International Development (USAID) to medical personnel in some 75 countries. Evaluations and recommendations were made that focused on needed changes in the determination of essential drugs on a country-wide basis and logistical requirements and determinants for developing countries around the world.

Upon graduation from UF with a Ph.D. my work experience other than in three small retail pharmacies was nil. When I accepted a position as a senior research scientist within the Department of Pharmaceutical Research and Development at the then Chas. Pfizer & Son (now Pfizer, Inc., since the mid-1960s), it was not for the difference in salary offered for a teaching position. As a result of my decision to proceed from graduate school to accept an offer to engage in pharmaceutical research in industry at that time, I became the first African American Ph.D. Senior Research Scientist at the then world's largest pharmaceutical manufacturer. My first pharmaceutical technology patent application was for Sustained Pharmaceutical Tablets (Patent 3,577,514) was filed on May 4, 1971, less than two years after I joined Pfizer, Inc.) and was awarded May 4, 1971.

In 1975, I was able to establish my own international pharmaceutical health care consulting operation, which enabled me to work with Federal agencies like the United States Agency for International Development, the World Health Organization, and the World Bank as well as the American Public Health Association, the John Snow Public Health Group, and Management Sciences for Health. I was also able to start a specialty pharmacy, manufacturing and wholesale pharmaceutical businesses (Universal Pharmaceuticals, Inc., and Universal Pharmaceutical Systems) which I operated for some 12 years before returning to Florida.

I left my highly successful career in pharmaceutical research and development at Pfizer, Inc. and became FAMU's Dean of the School of Pharmacy on August 1, 1969, when the school was on probation by the national accreditation agency, the American Council on Pharmaceutical Education (ACPE). At the time, I was the youngest pharmacy dean in the country. My planned tenure as professor of pharmacy and Dean was always temporary. I had chosen a career in industrial pharmacy – more specifically pharmaceutical product research and development – and had all intentions of returning to the pharmaceutical industry after the School of Pharmacy had reclaimed its full national accreditation, dramatically restructured its pharmacy curriculum incorporating, and had begun to acquire significant increased amounts of state, federal and external funding.

After we had achieved our principal and considerable goals with substantial facility, financial and broad-based alumni and public support, I was ready and had all intentions of returning to the pharmaceutical manufacturing industry. However, our achievements became more broadly known nationally and now my raised profile as a national leader in pharmaceutical education, enabled me to be elected to the position as first Secretary-Treasurer of the Council of Deans of the American Association of Colleges of Pharmacy, State Director for the American College of Apothecaries, and member of an essential committee of the American Institute of the History of Pharmacy, etc.

I also worked closely with FAMU senior pharmacy student, John Scrivens, Jr., and supported his, and Howard University's senior pharmacy student Sharon Roquemore's efforts in forming the initial Student National Pharmaceutical Association (SNPhA) with their then chaperone, Rosalyn C. Cain (now Dr. Rosalyn C. King). I fully supported this effort by drafting the first by-laws for the SNPhA and hosting the organizers in Tallahassee, FL.

As we were completing the FAMU School of Pharmacy move into its first new and dedicated facility, the Dyson Pharmacy Building, named after the late African American state legislator, I was able to complete and formalize the National Pharmaceutical Foundation (NPF), which was incorporated in Washington, DC in early 1973. Because of the glaring need for such an organization, I began the effort during my final few months at FAMU with the eager assists of Ramona D. McCarthy, Rosalyn C. King, and the deans of the four historically African American colleges of pharmacy – Howard University, where I had just, assumed the deanship of the college as of January 1, 1973; as well as FAMU, Xavier University of Louisiana, and Texas Southern University.

The National Pharmaceutical Foundation (NPF) had as its principal objectives the promotion of equal opportunity for African American and other minority pharmacists in education, employment and entrepreneurship. In pursuance of those objectives, the NPF:

1. Initially sponsored the new Student National Pharmaceutical Association (SNPhA) for several years before the National Pharmaceutical Association (NPhA) associated its national organization with this student group.
2. Raised funds from the pharmaceutical industry and various foundations to fund scholarships for needy minority pharmacy students and the SNPhA;
3. Publicly recognized the achievements and contributions of African American pharmacists in the following areas:
    a. National pharmacy association leadership: recognized *Mary Munson Runge,* first woman to head up the APhA.
    b. Legislative and political leadership: recognized *Mickey Leland* (D-Texas), the first pharmacist to Chair, the Congressional Black Caucus, and *Byron Rumsford* (D-Calif.)
    c. Presidents of State Boards of Pharmacy: *Albert Hopkins*, first African American President of the Texas State Board of Pharmacy.
4. Sponsored several national symposia on *Progress and Problems of Black Pharmacists in America.*

I certainly hope that this background information will provide some further valuable insights into the developmental history of education of African American pharmacists in the U.S. by contributing to the increased detail and accuracy of this most valuable document.

Ira Charles Robinson, Ph.D., R.Ph.
Former FAMU Dean and Professor of Pharmacy
Former Howard University Dean and Professor of Pharmacy

Appendix A

Early African American Pharmacy Graduates and Students from Predominantly White Universities in the North: 1895–1963

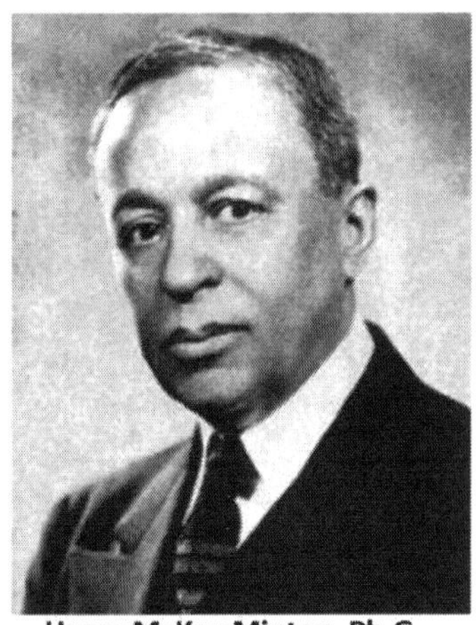

Henry McKee Minton, Ph.G.
Philadelphia College of Pharmacy
1895

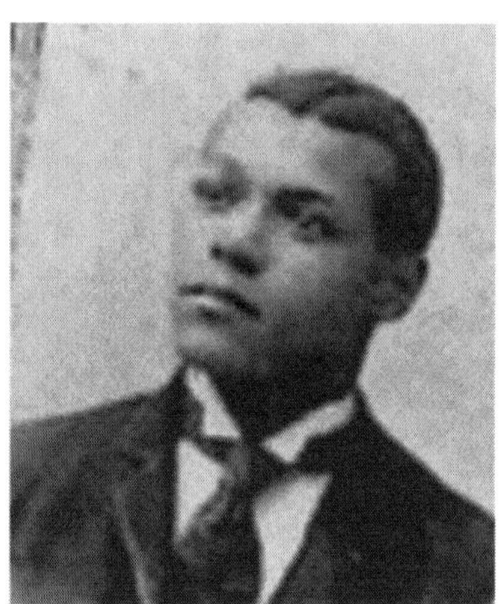

Arthur K. Lawrence, Ph.G.
Ohio State University
1897

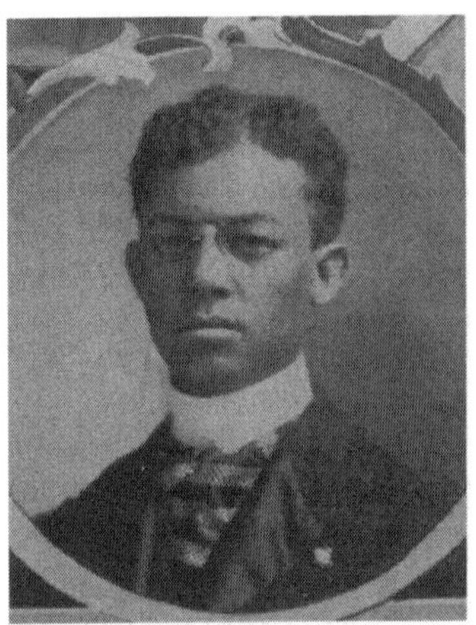

John Allen McFall, PD
Philadelphia College of Pharmacy
1899

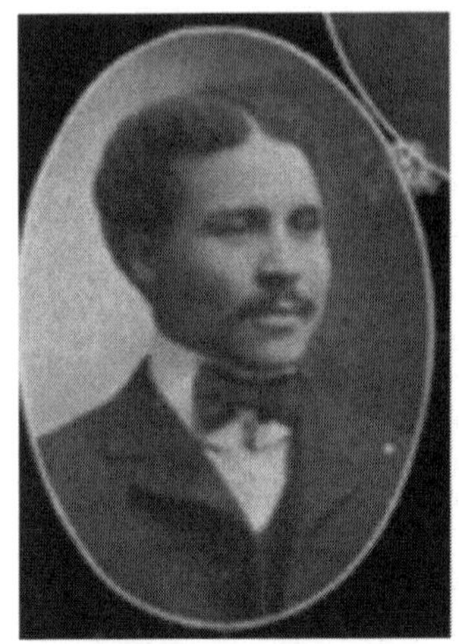

Edward W. Thompson, Ph.G.
University of Iowa
1907

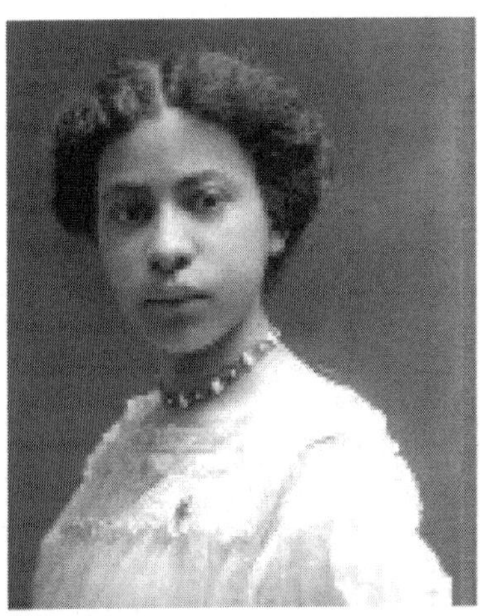

Anna Louise James, Ph.G.
Brooklyn College of Pharmacy
1908

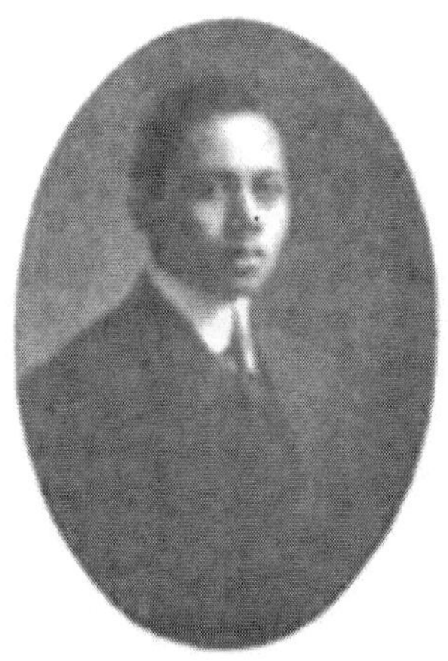

Augustus A. Williams, Ph.C. B.S.
University of Michigan
1908

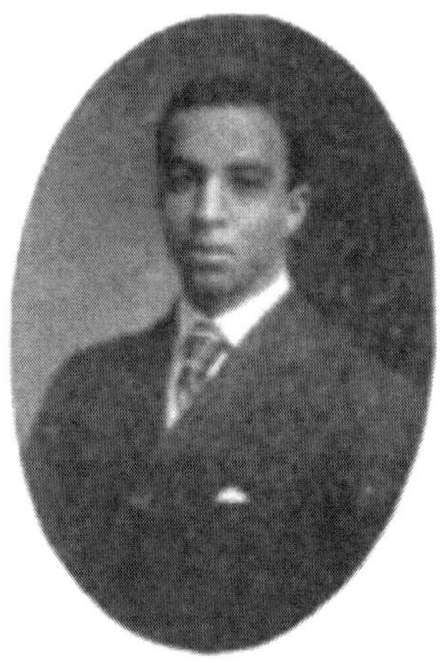

Norris A. Dobson, Ph.G., B.S.
University of Michigan
1908, 1910

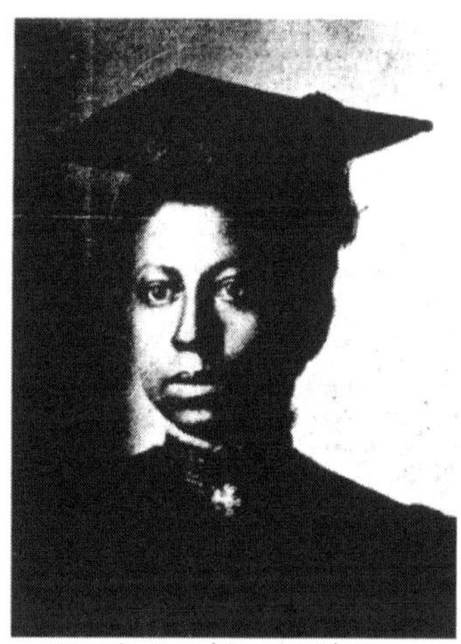

Hattie Hutchinson, Ph.G.
Highland Park College of Pharmacy
1908

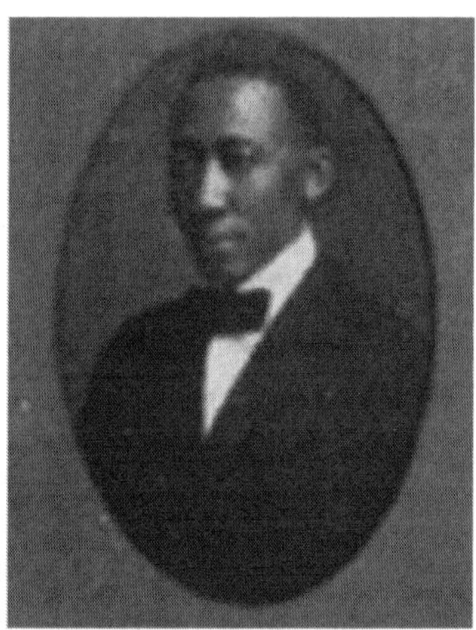

Nicholas Alfred Garfield Diggs, Ph.C.
University of Michigan
1910

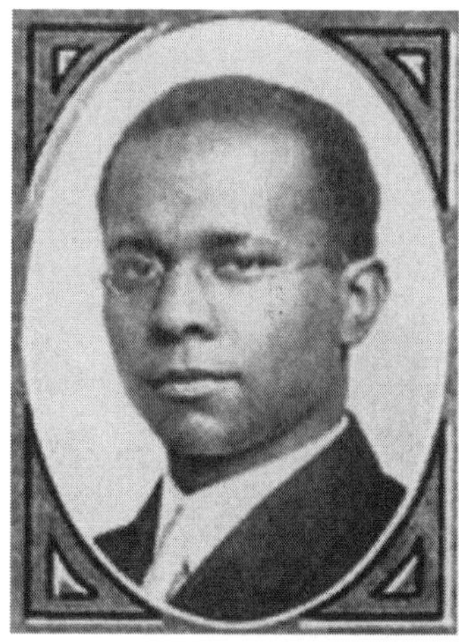

Mathieu Virgil Boutte, Ph.G., Ph.C.
University of Illinois
1911

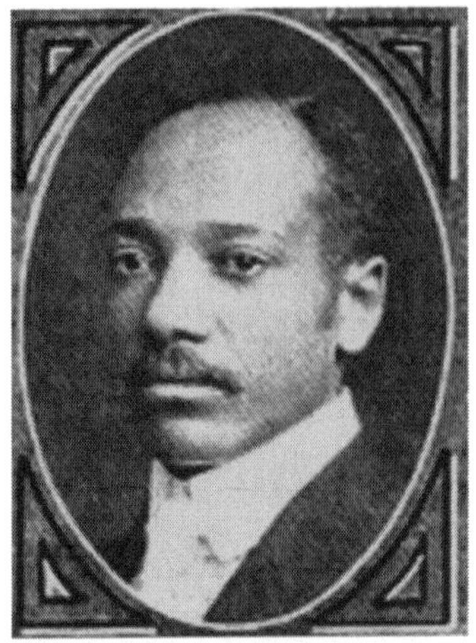

Solomon Leroy Lee, Ph.G.
University of Illinois
1911

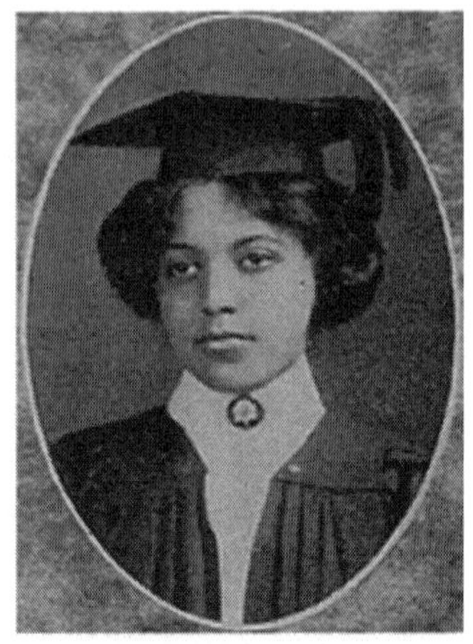

Alice Augusta Ball, Ph.C., B.S.
University of Washington
1912

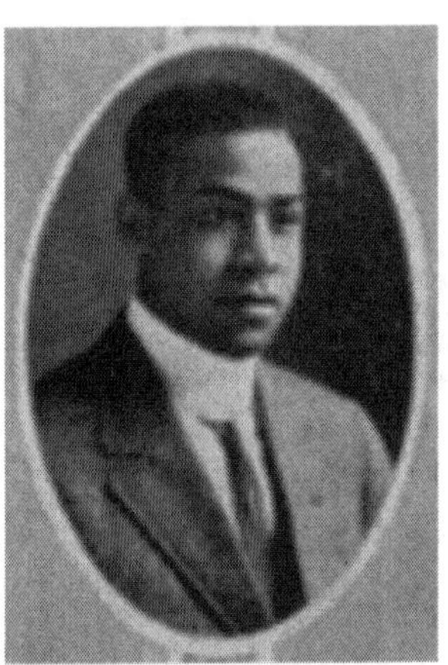

Ewell E. Clemons, Ph.C.
University of Michigan
1912

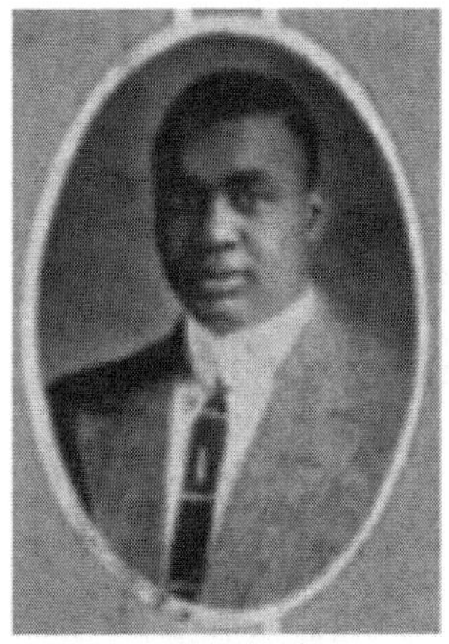

James H. Hilburn, Ph.C.
University of Michigan
1912

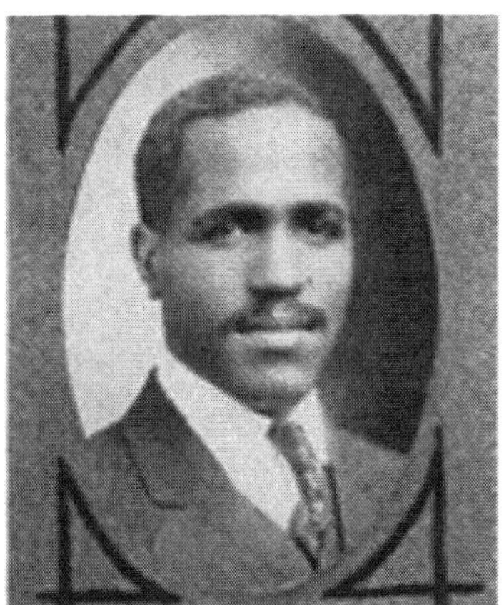

William Sylvester White, Ph.G.
University of Illinois
1912

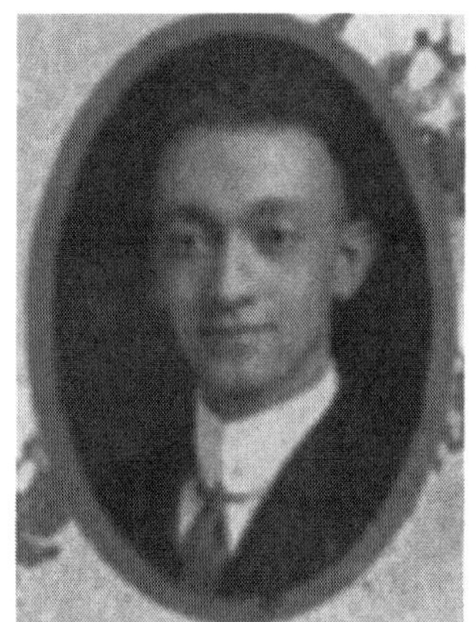

Basie S. Braxton, Ph.C.
University of Michigan
1913

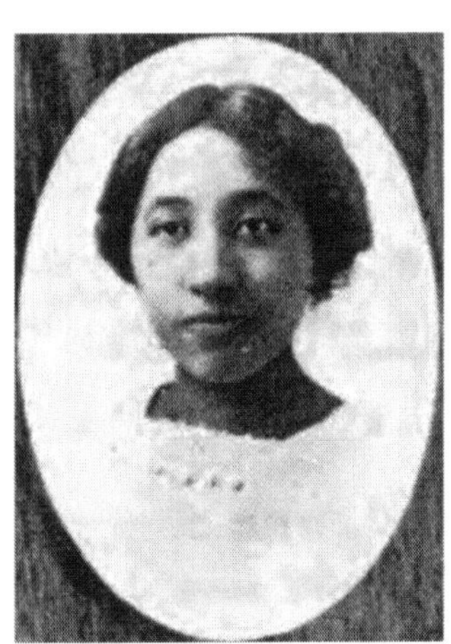

Fannie Jamison, Ph.G.
Ohio State University
1913

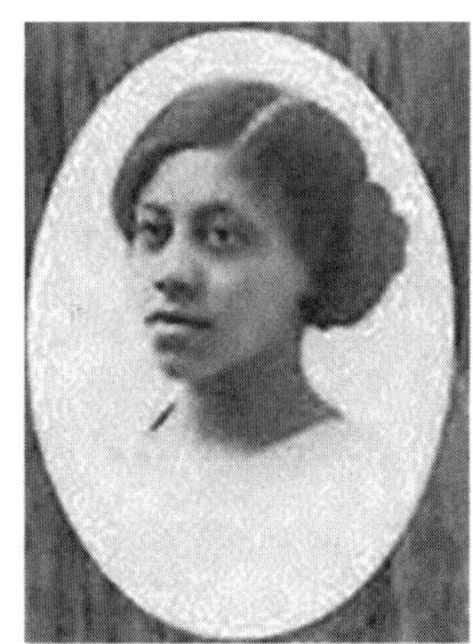

Florence M. Burns, Ph.G.
Ohio State University
1913

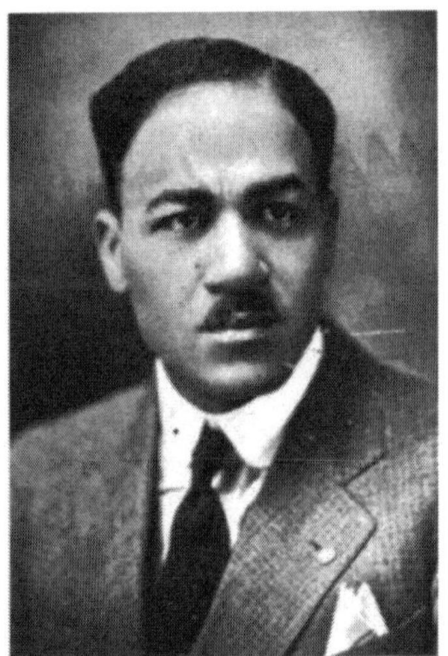

Raymond W. Cannon, Ph.B.
University of Minnesota
1913

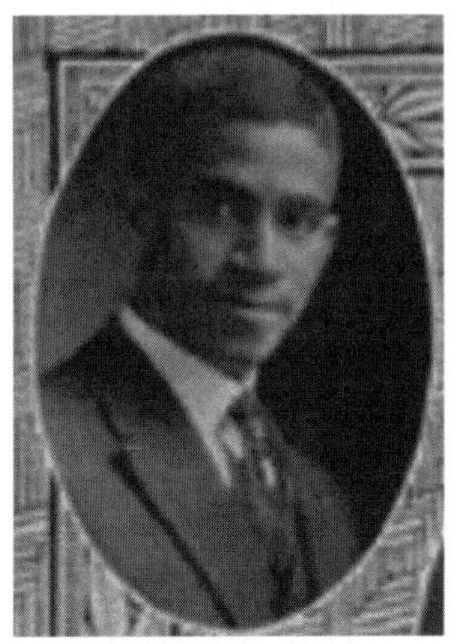

Curtis F. Jenkins, Ph.C.
University of Michigan
1914

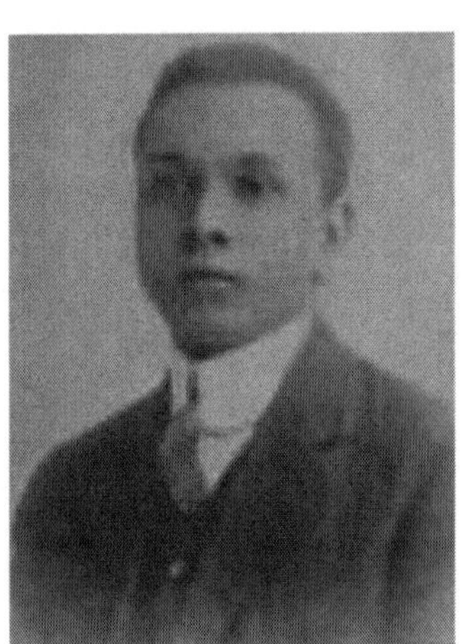

William Wyatt Stewart, Ph.G.
University of Pittsburgh
1914

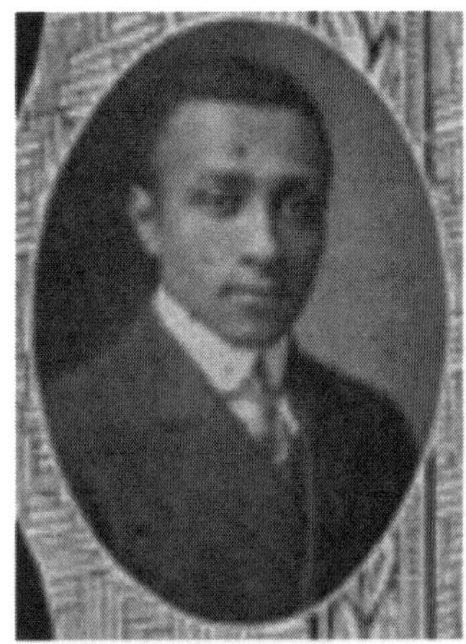

Max W. Johnson, Ph.C.
University of Michigan
1914

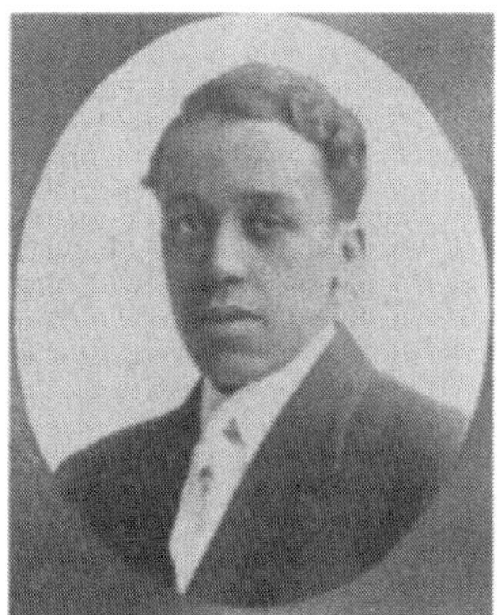

Marion Harris Tanner, Ph.G.
University of Pittsburgh
1915

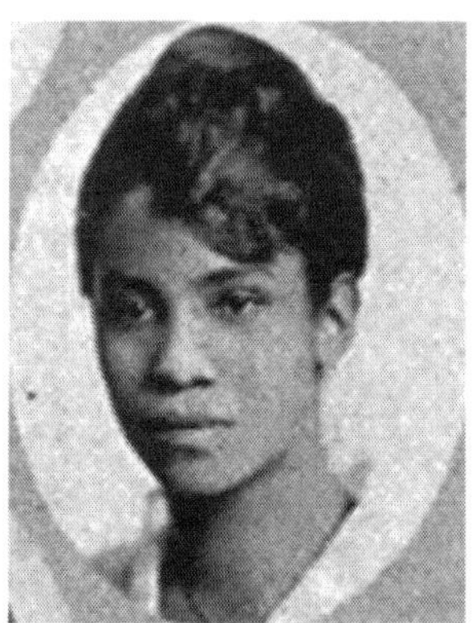

Olive D. Howard, Ph.G.
University of Minnesota
1915

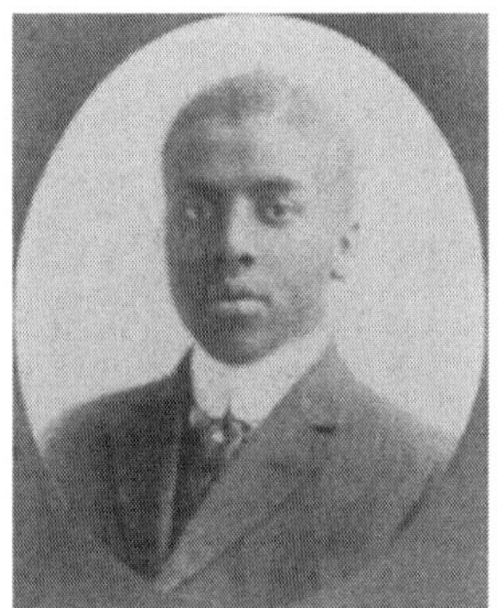

Stanley Wilbert Jefferson, Ph.G.
University of Pittsburgh
1915

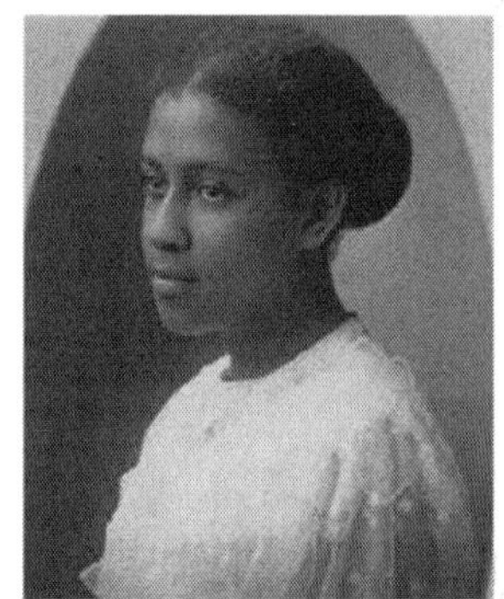

Rosamond Alice Guinn, Ph.G.
Massachusetts College of Pharmacy
1915

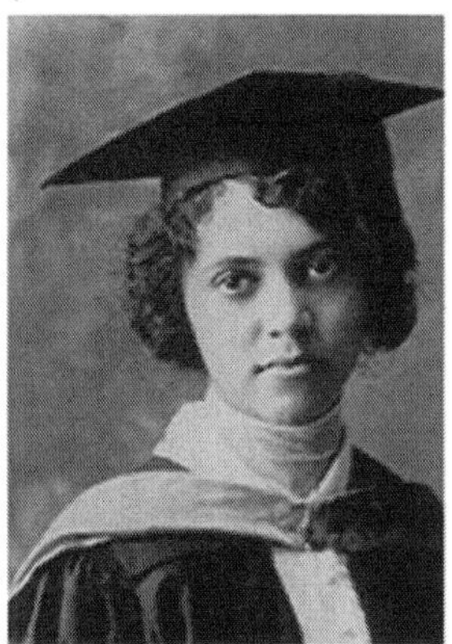

Alice Augustus Ball, M.S.
University of Hawaii
1915

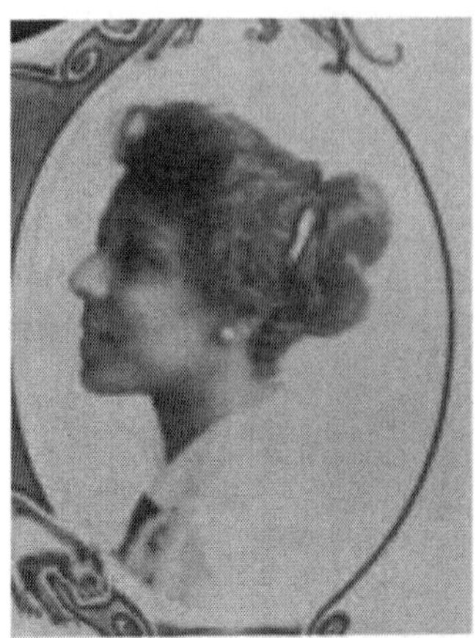

Charlotte Louisa Austin, P.C.
University of Pittsburgh
1916

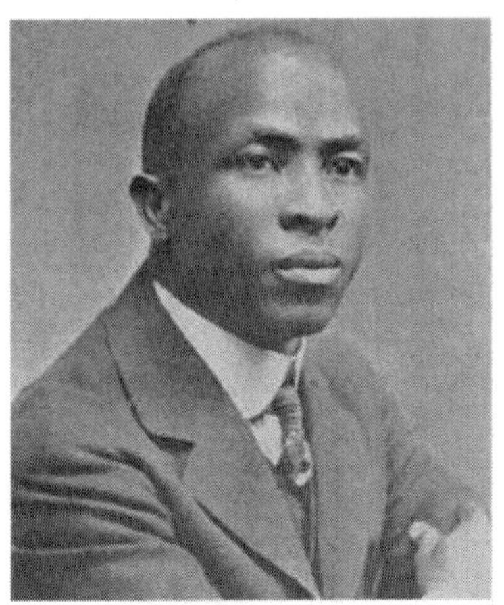

Walter Lee Brandon, Ph.G.
Temple University
1916

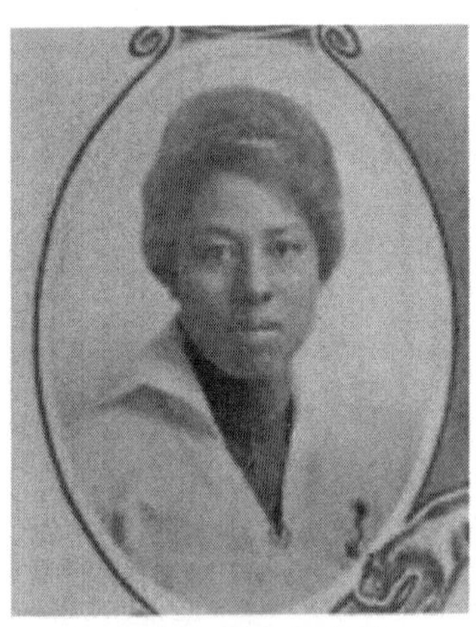

Ella Phillips Myers, Ph.G.
University of Pittsburgh
1916

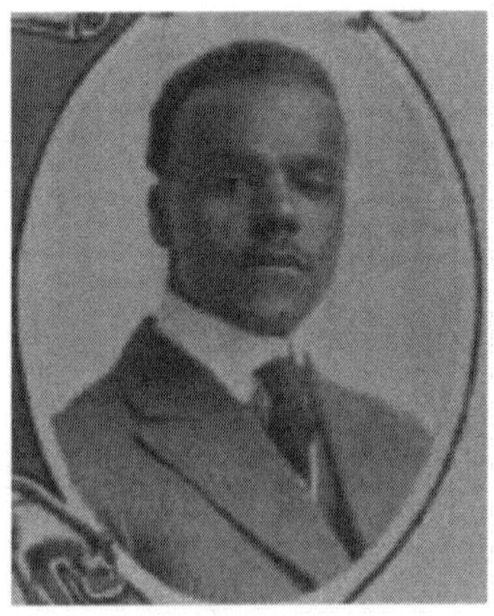

George G. Williams, Ph.G.
University of Pittsburgh
1916

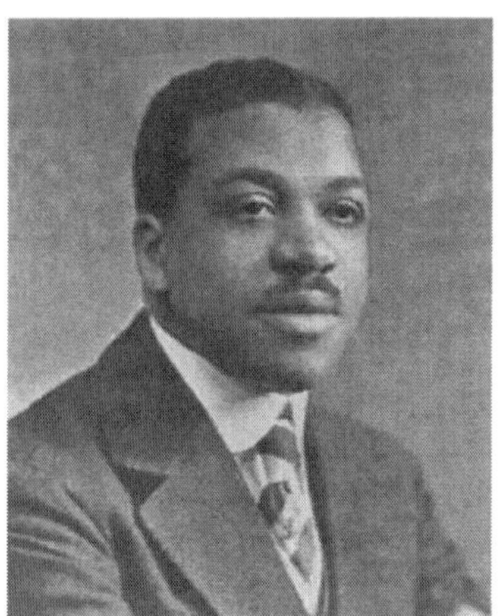

Raymond H. Rodgers, Ph.G.
Temple University
1916

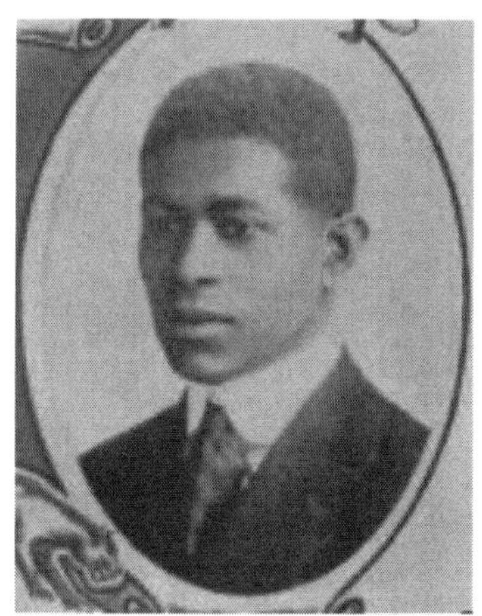

Richard B. Carter, Ph.G.
University of Pittsburgh
1916

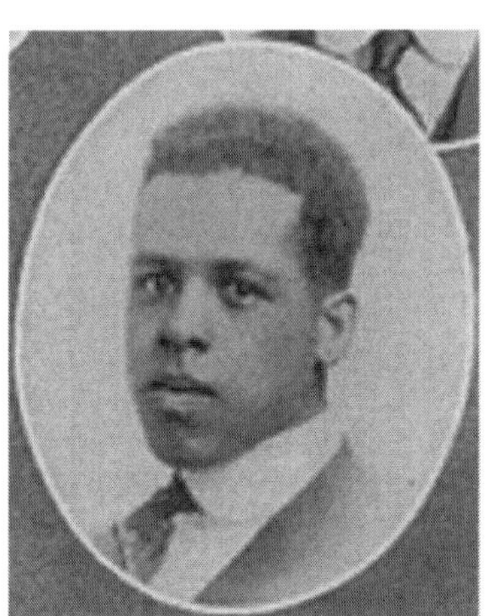

Eugene Langston, Ph.C.
Northwestern University
1917

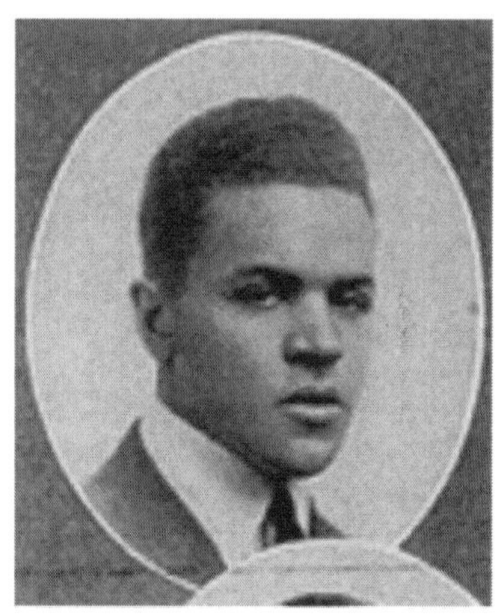

Gerald Clifton Bunn, Ph.G.
Northwestern University
1917

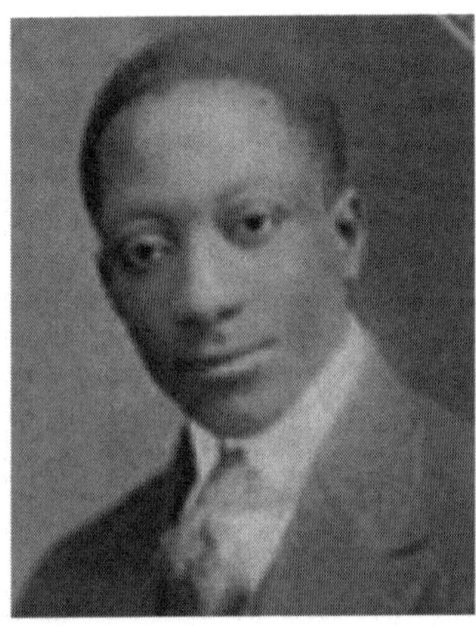

Antonio F. Lalondily St Clara, Ph.G.
Ohio Northern University
1918

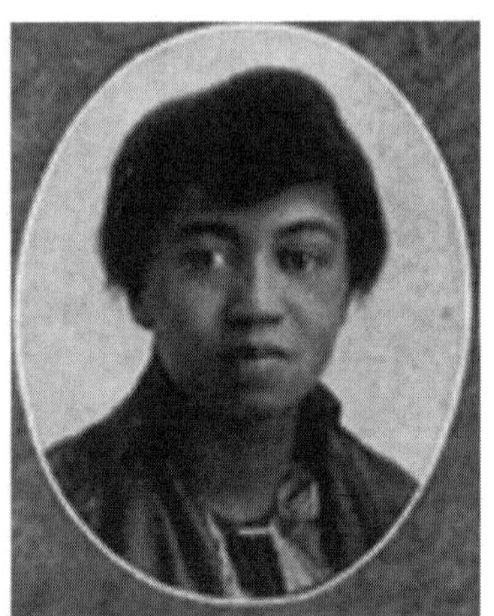

Mildred C. Gunn, Ph.G.
University of Pittsburgh
1918

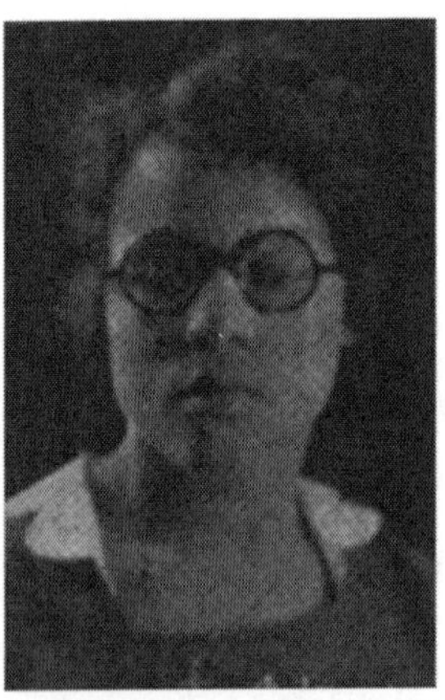

Anna P. J. Comegys, Ph.G., Phar.D.
Temple University
1919

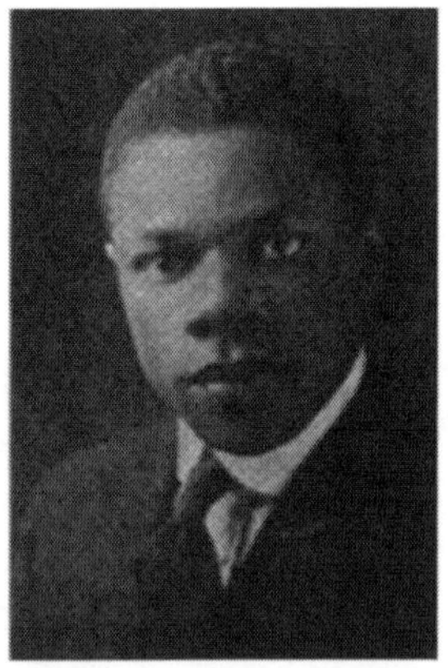

George T. Hunter, Ph.G.
Temple University
1920

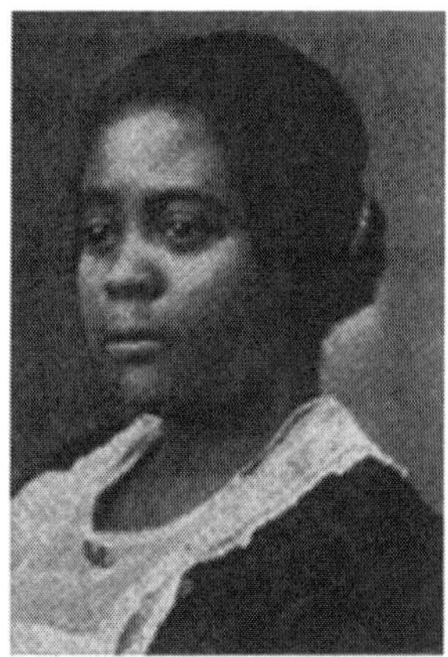

Gelia V. Harris, Ph.G.
Temple University
1920

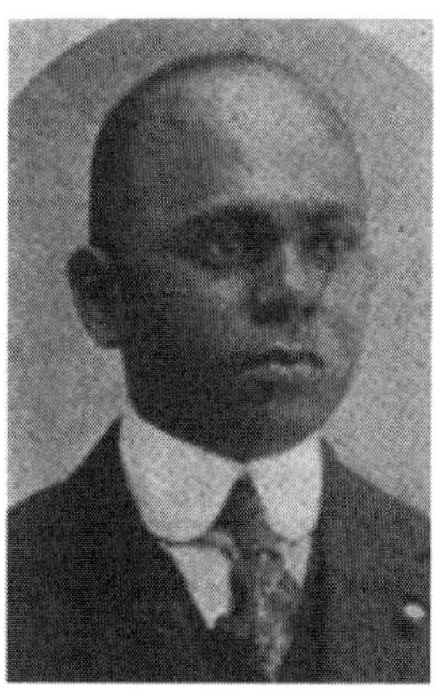

John H. Lassiter, Ph.G.
Temple University
1920

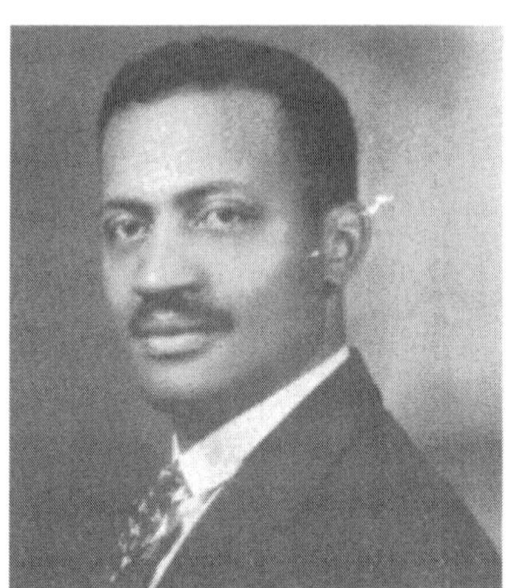

Wiley C. Baines, Ph.C.
University of Minnesota
1921

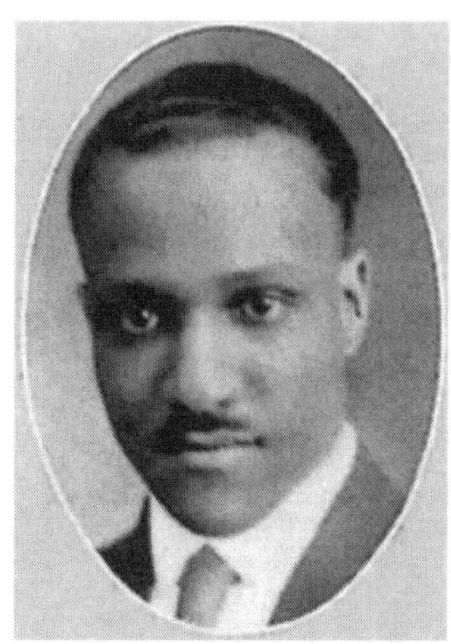

Spotswood McKinley Green, Ph.G.
Ohio State University
1922

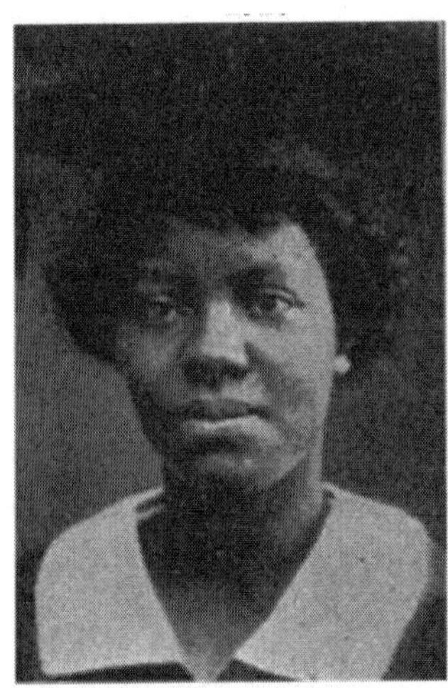

Alice E. Bunce, Ph. G.
New Jersey College of Pharmacy
1923

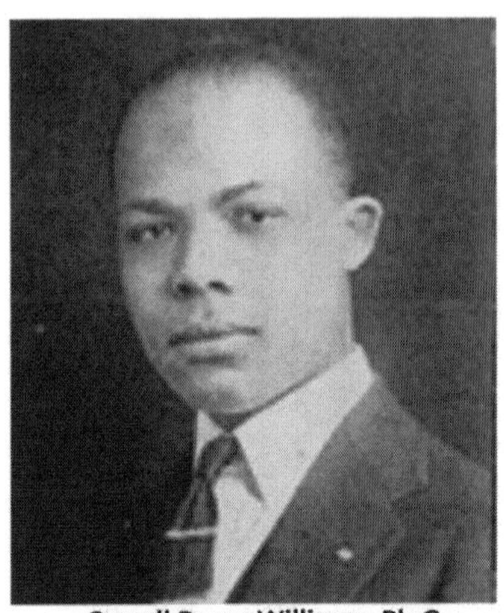

Carroll Burns Williams, Ph.G.
Massachusetts College of Pharmacy
1923

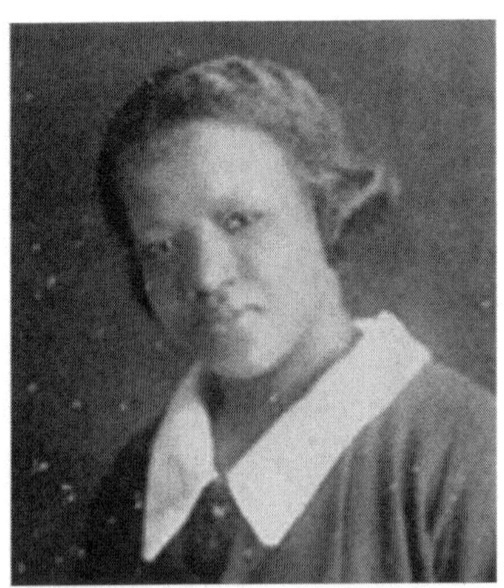

Estelle Marie Anderson, Ph.G.
Massachusetts College of Pharmacy
1923

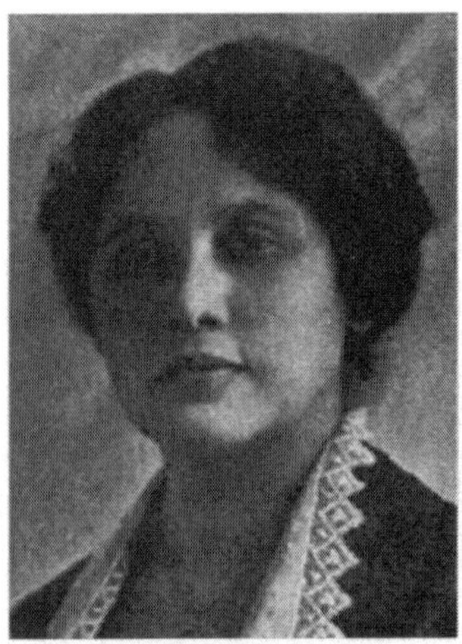

Etnah Rochon Boutte, Ph.G.
City College of New York
1923

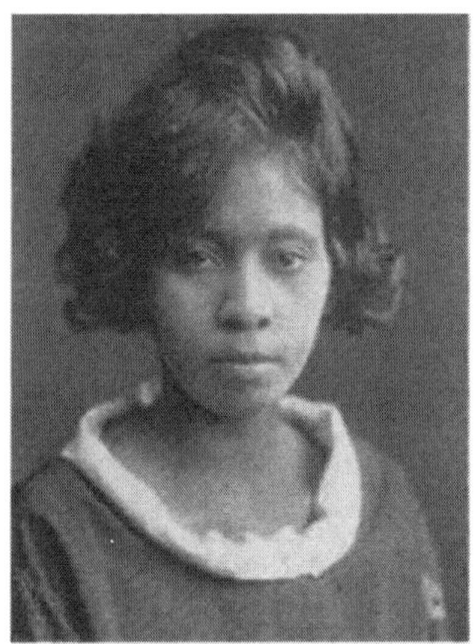

Efie Nevers, Ph.G.
Philadelphia College of Pharmacy
1923

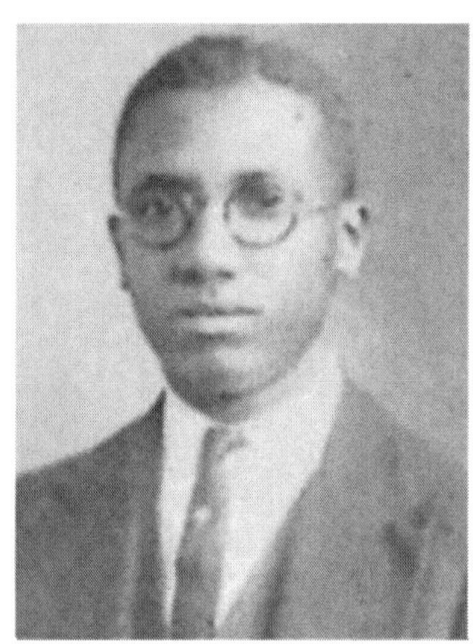

Percy Willard Giddings, Ph.G.
Ohio State University
1923

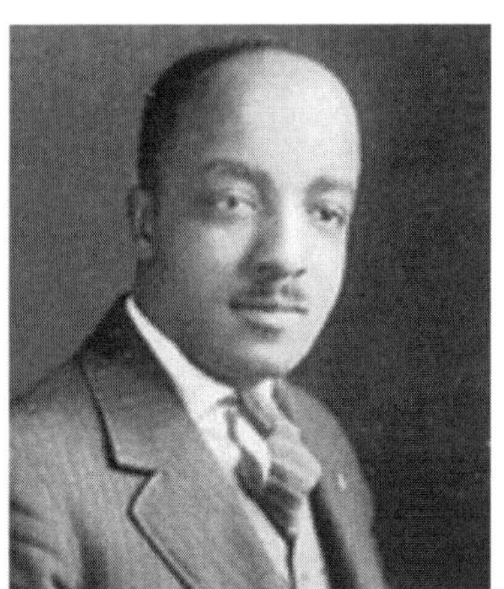

Robert Lloyd Graham, Ph.G.
Massachusetts College of Pharmacy
1923

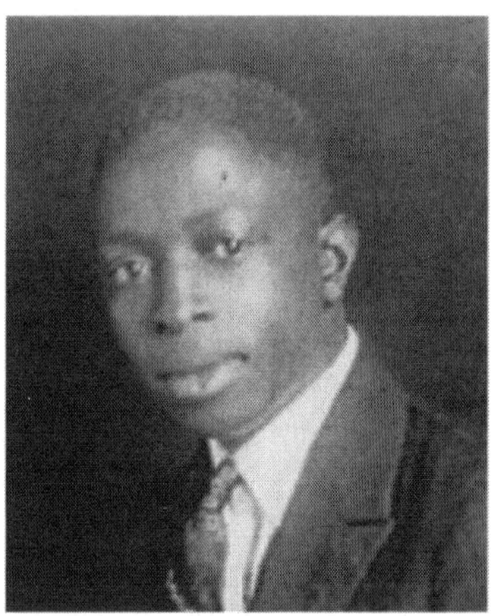

Tracy McClinton Walton, Ph.G.
Massachusetts College of Pharmacy
1923

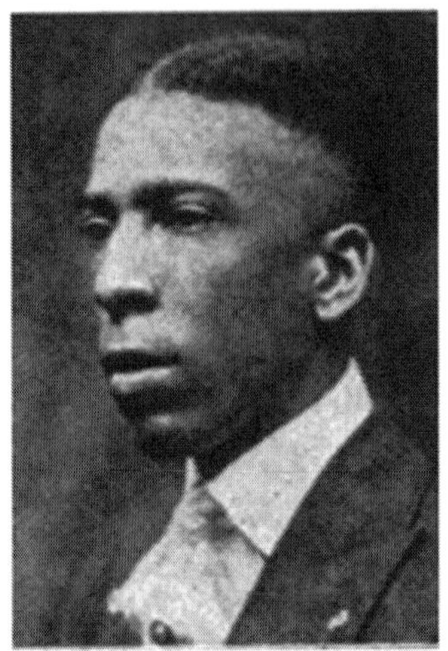

Scott A. McCoy, Ph.G
University of Pittsburgh
1923

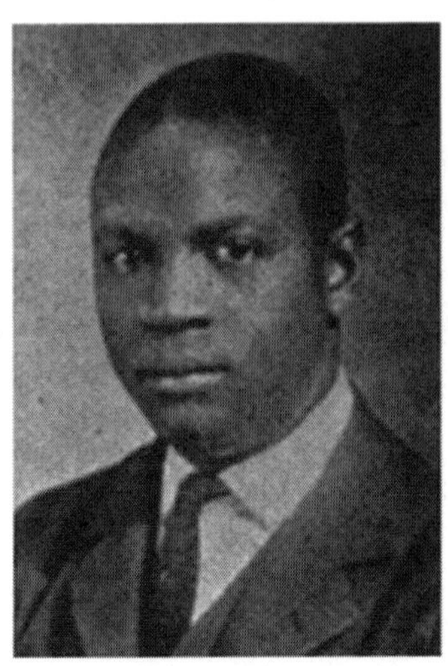

Cyrus T. L. Dabney, Ph.G.
Columbia University
1923

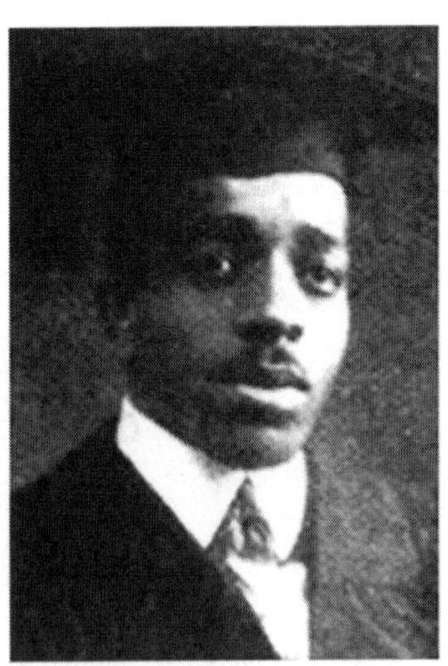

E.D. Giggetts, Ph.G.
New Jersey College of Pharmacy
1923

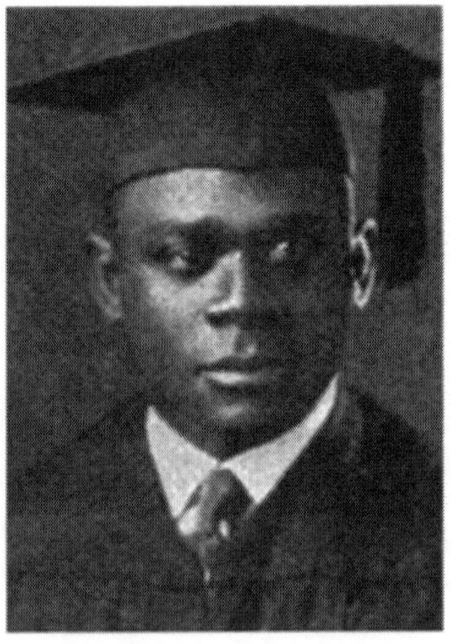

Joseph Jennings, Ph.G.
Columbia University
1923

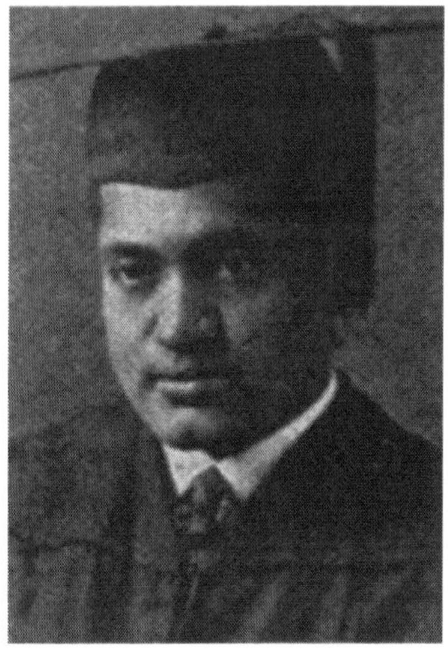

Wallace S. Hayes, Ph.G.
Columbia University
1923

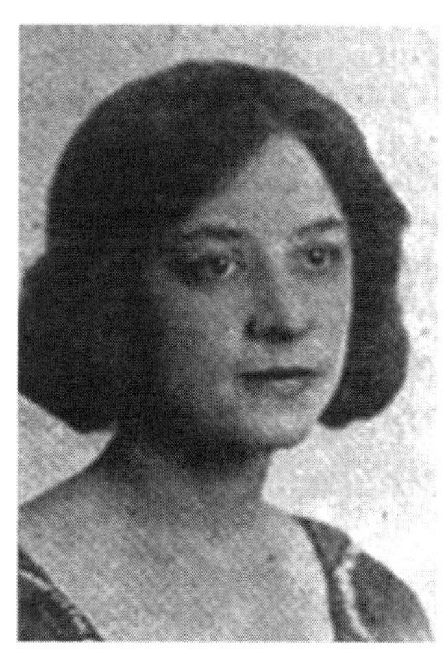

Coty Johnson, Ph.G.
University of Southern California
1923

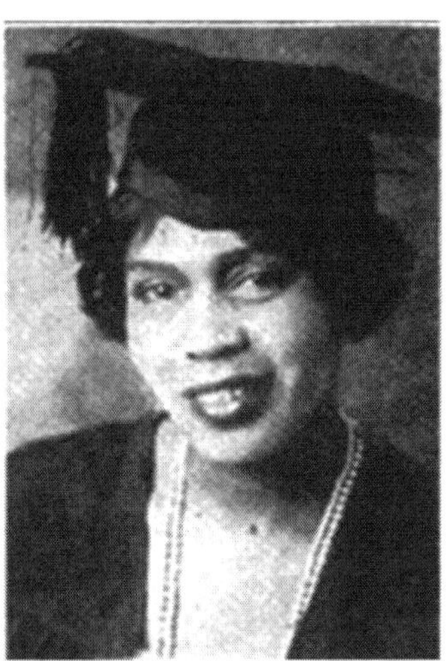

Emily B. Childress, Ph.G.
University of Southern California
1923

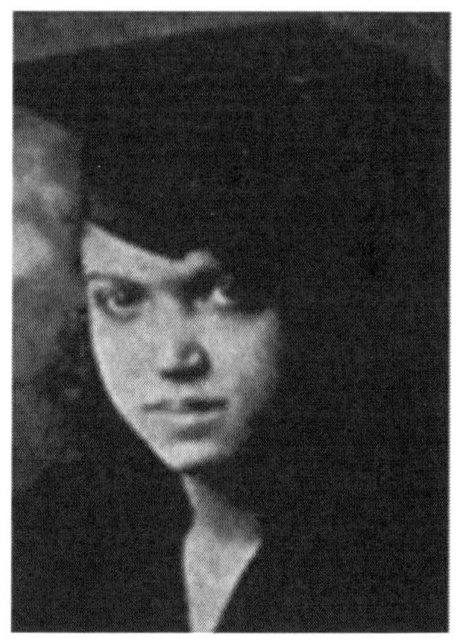

Ursula Pruitt, Ph.G.
University of Southern California
1923

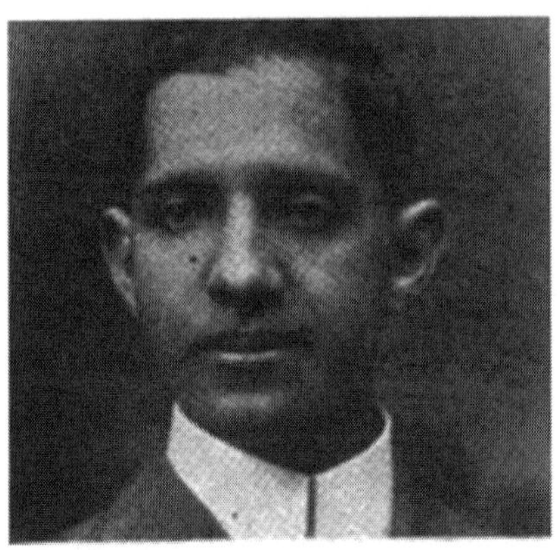

Benjamin A. Quarles, Ph.C., Ph.G.
University of Pittsburgh
1923

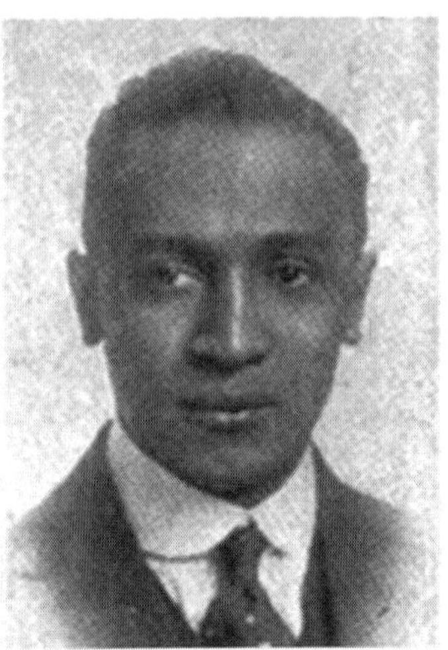

Frederick D. Inge, Ph.C.
University of Minnesota
1923

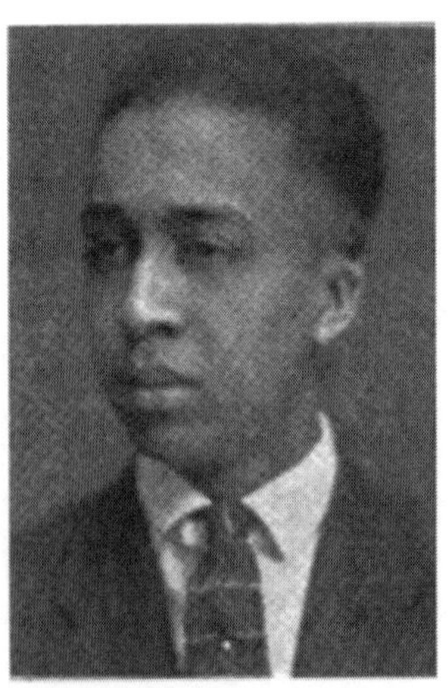

M. C. Amos, Ph.C.
University of Cincinnati
1923

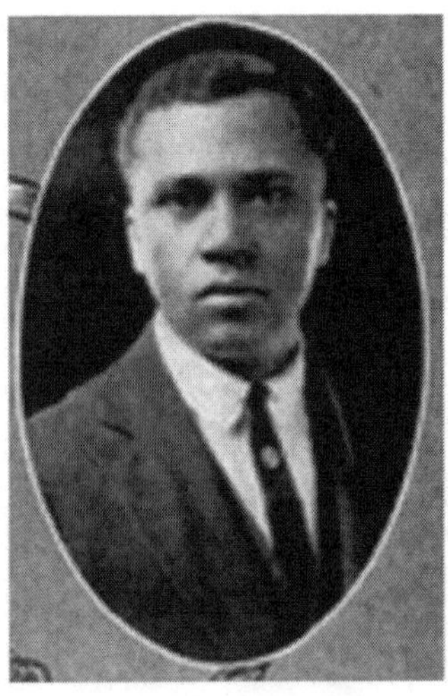

Olfred O. Nash, Ph.G.
Purdue University
1923

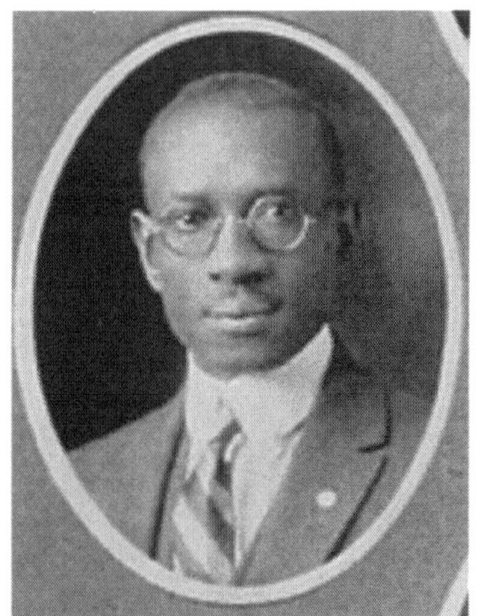

John D. Ammon, Ph.G.
City College of New York
1924

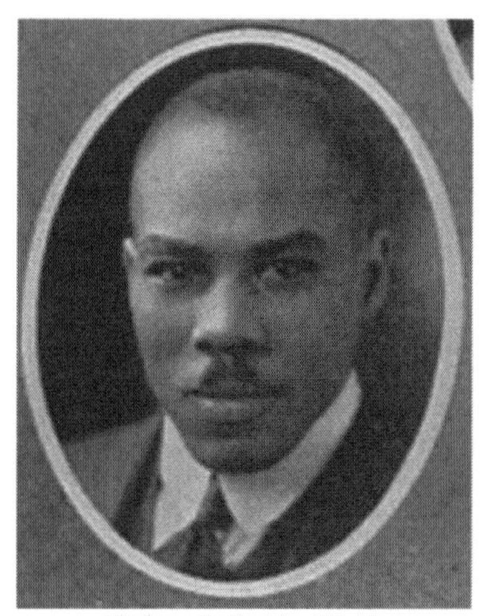

Walter F. Battle, Ph.G.
City College of New York
1924

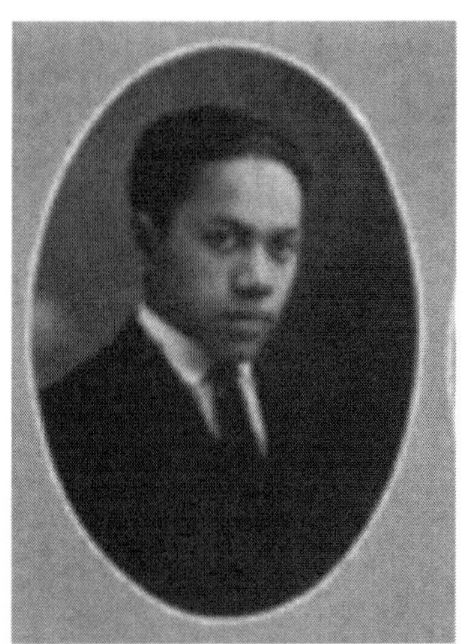

William S. Avery, Ph.G.
University of Iowa
1924

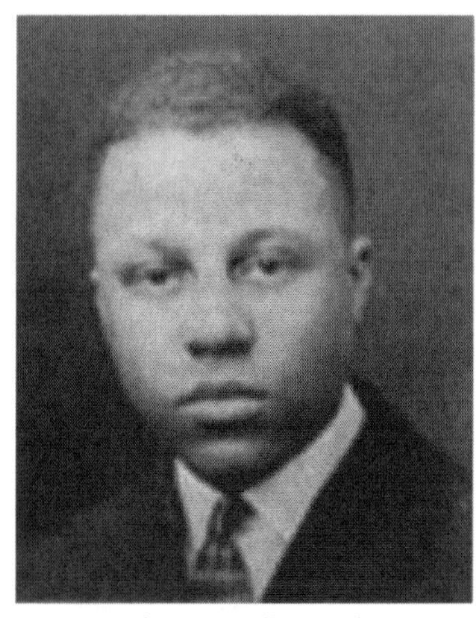

Cornelius K. Wilkins, Ph.G.
Case Western Reserve University
1925

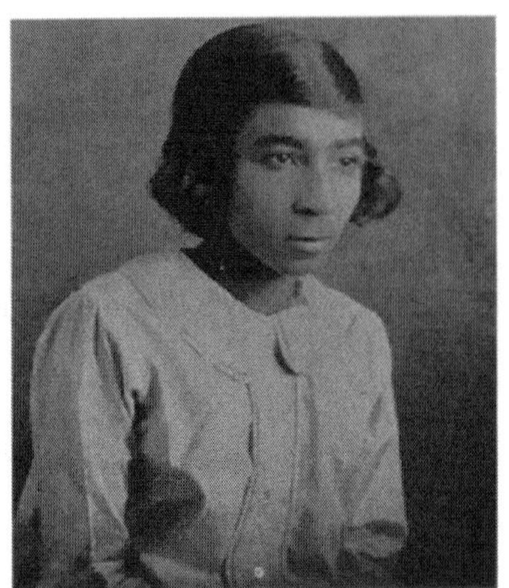

Frances Moses, Ph.G.
Temple University
1926

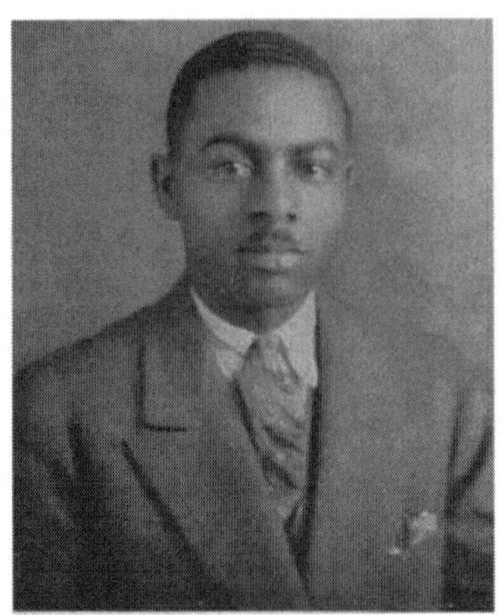

George M. White, Ph.G.
Temple University
1926

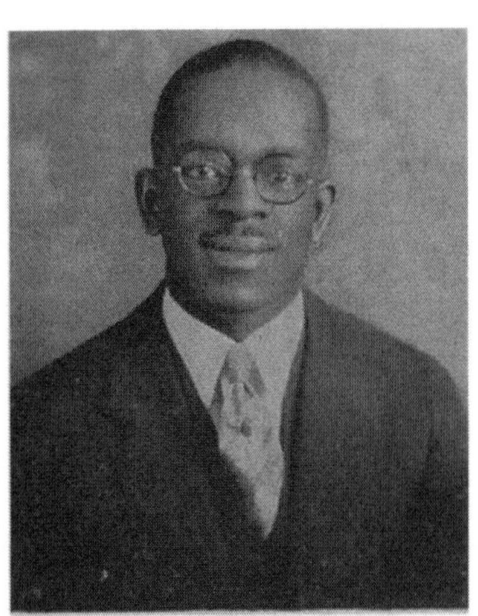

John Loper, Ph.G.
Temple University
1926

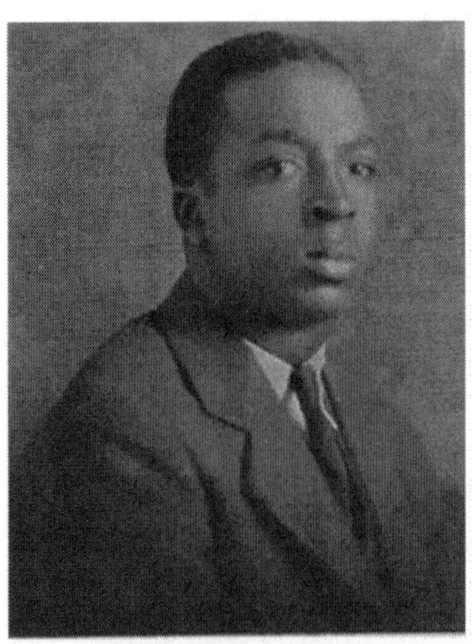

Maris Wesley, Ph.G.
Temple University
1926

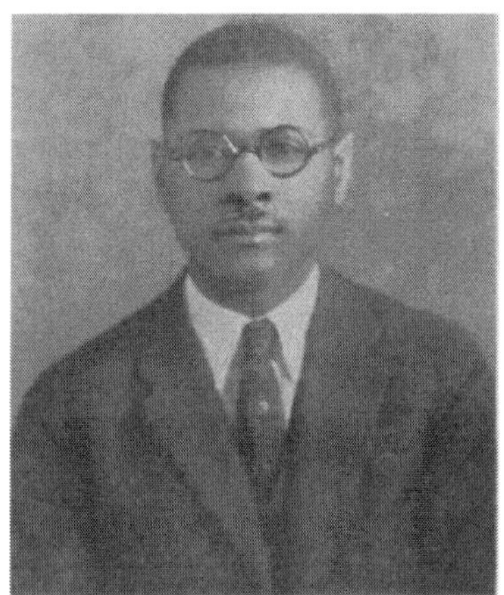

Paul Foster, Ph.G.
Temple University
1926

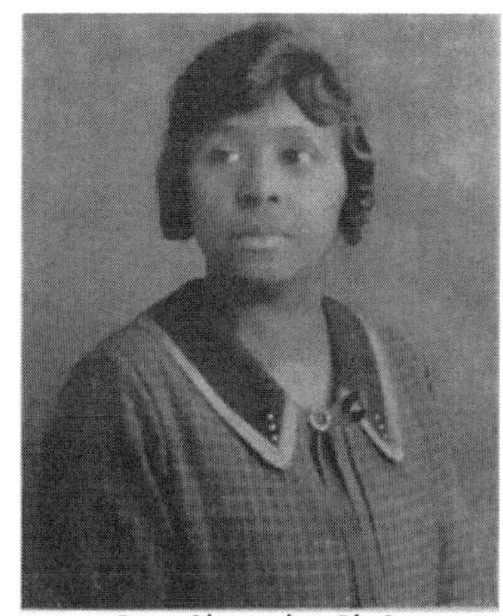

Rosa Alexander, Ph.G.
Temple University
1926

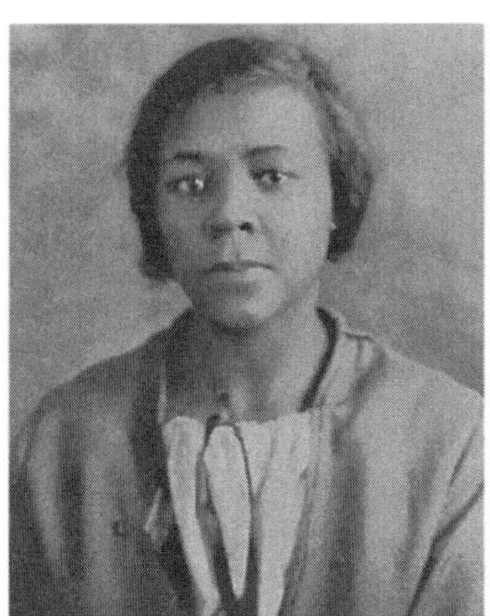

Ruth Downing, Ph.G.
Temple University
1926

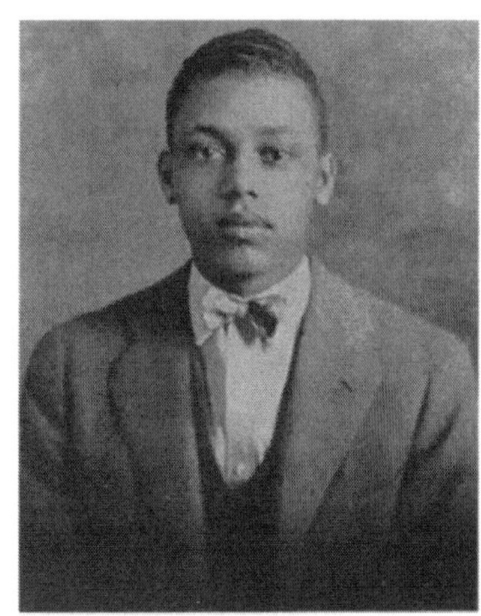

William Dean, Ph.G.
Temple University
1926

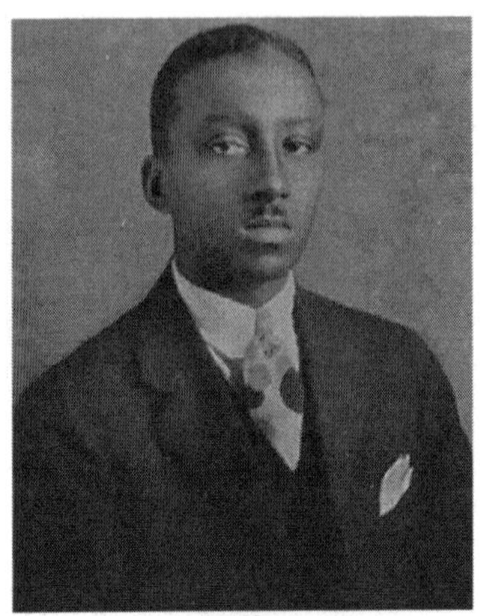

John F. Williams, Ph.G.
Temple University
1926

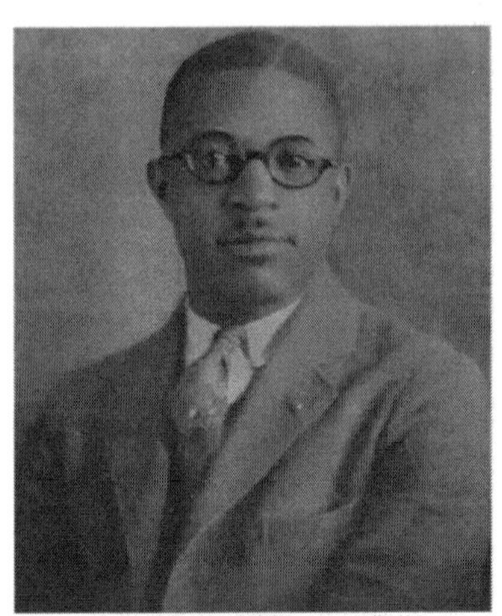

Joseph M. Williams, Ph.G.
Temple University
1926

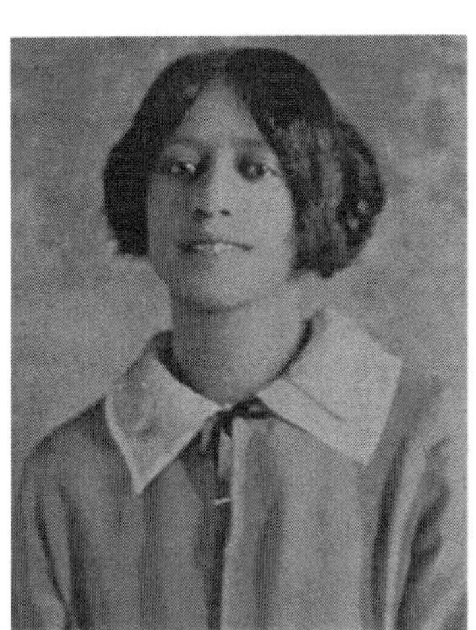

Audrey Gray, Ph.G.
Temple University
1926

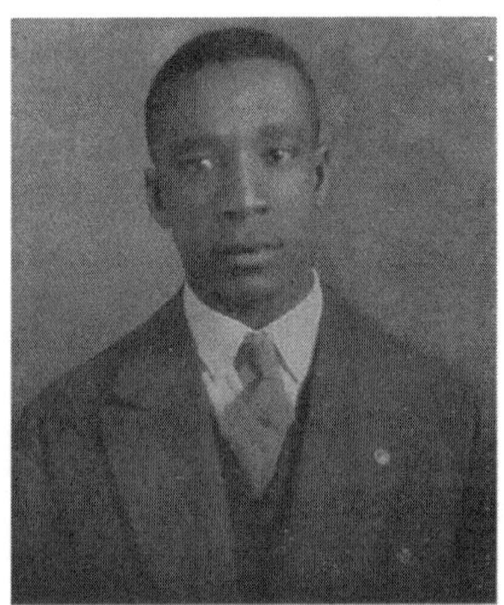

Benjamin Warner, Ph.G.
Temple University
1926

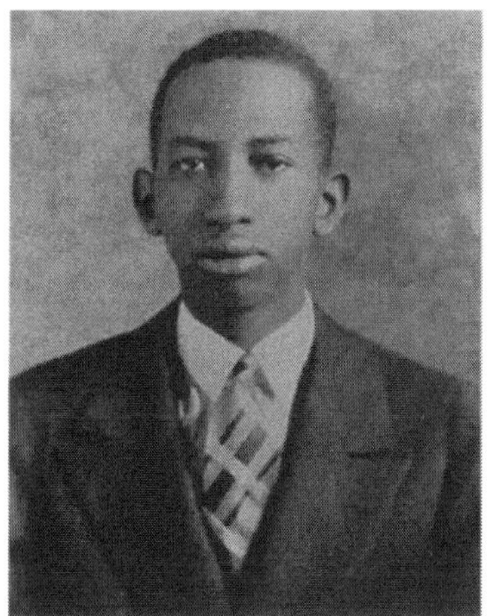

Henry H. Winters, Ph.G.
Temple University
1926

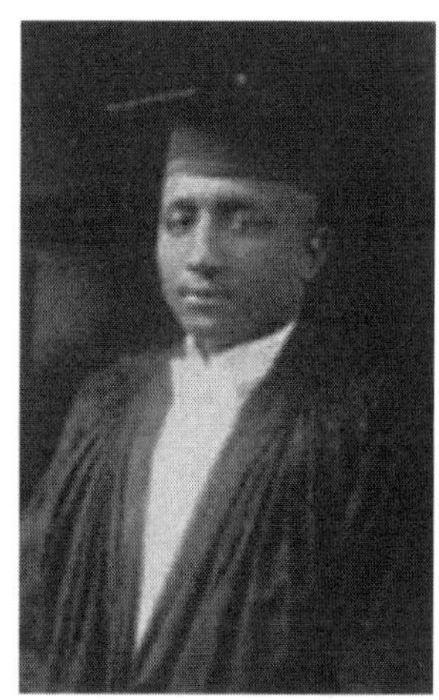

Aaron A. Larry, Ph.G.
Detroit College of Pharmacy
1926

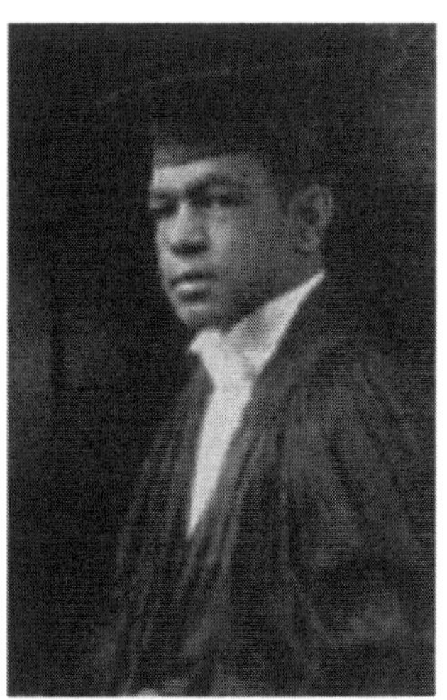

Berner D. Johnson, Ph.G.
Detroit College of Pharmacy
1926

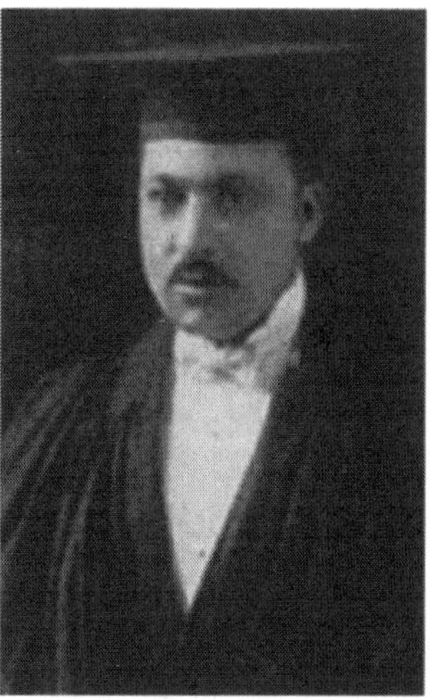

James Benson, Ph.G.
Detroit College of Pharmacy
1926

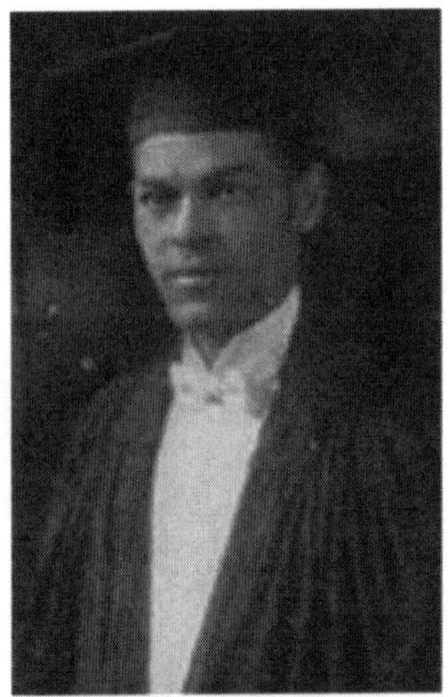

Leo Robinson, Ph.G.
Detroit College of Pharmacy
1926

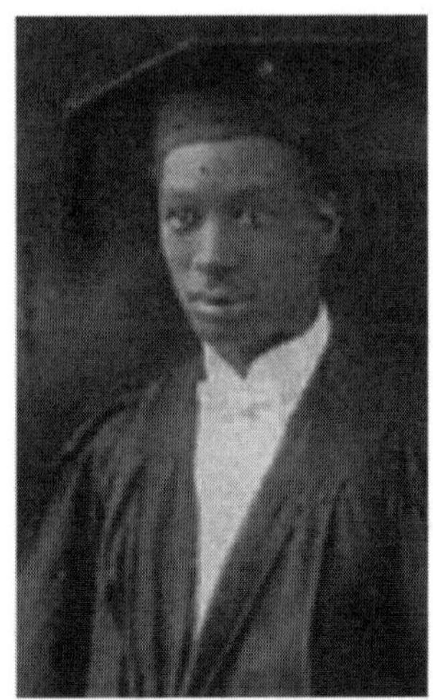

Samuel A. Hall, Ph.G.
Detroit College of Pharmacy
1926

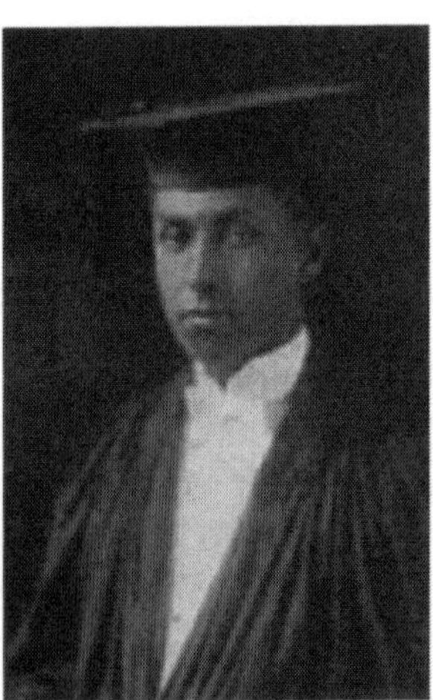

Sherman Hardiman, Ph.G.
Detroit College of Pharmacy
1926

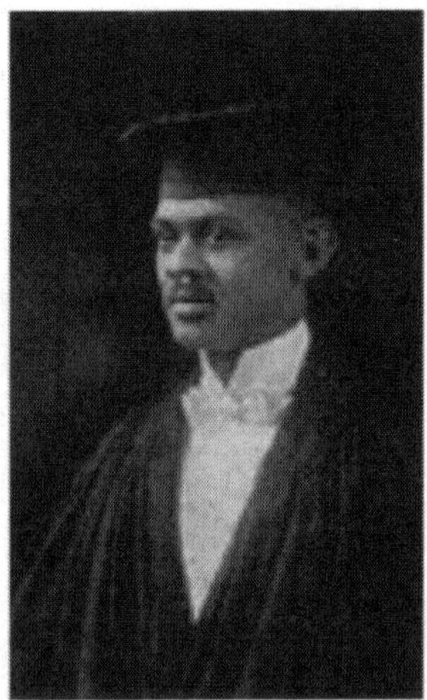

Snowflake Grigsby, Ph.G.
Detroit College of Pharmacy
1926

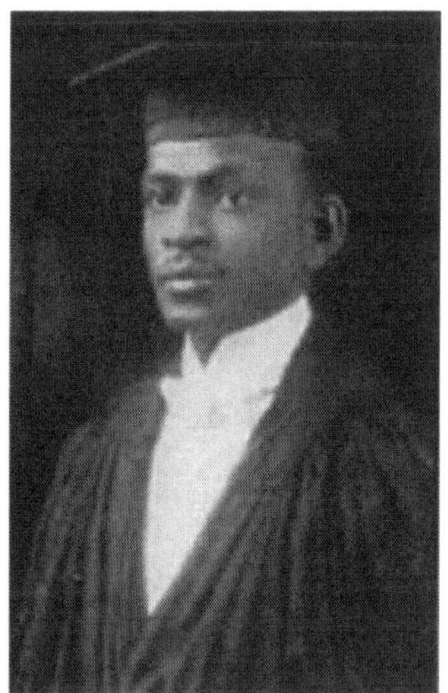

Talley E. Wells, Ph.G.
Detroit College of Pharmacy
1926

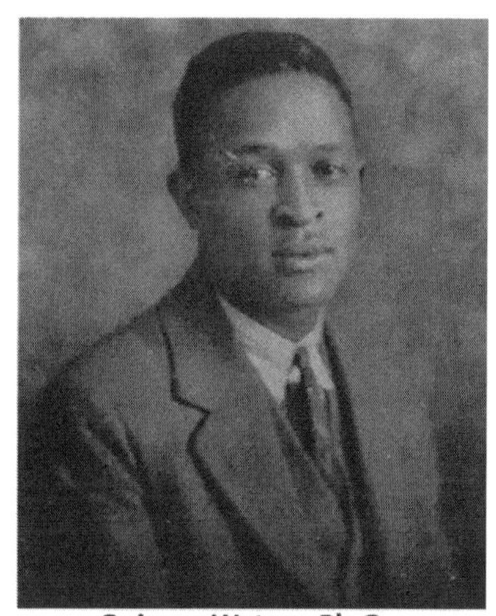

Quincey Waters, Ph.G.
Temple University
1926

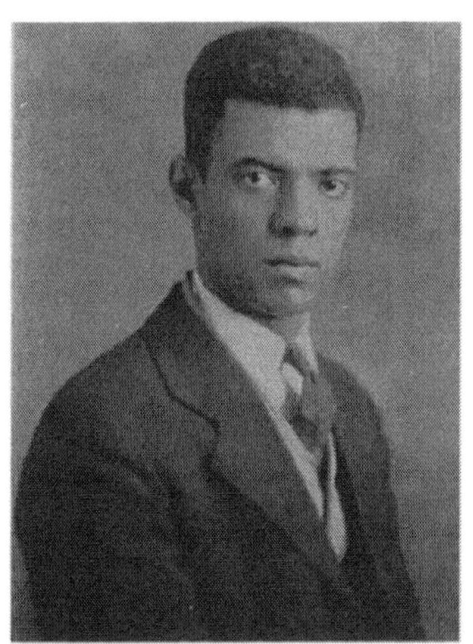

Theodore Brown, Ph.G.
Temple University
1926

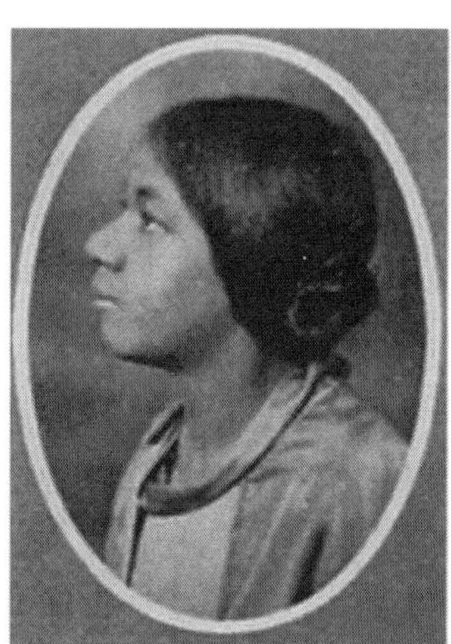

Vivian Irvin, Ph.G.
City College of New York
1927

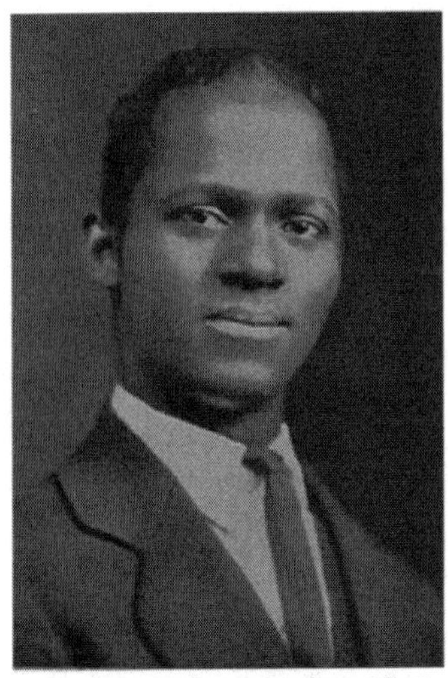

Charles Herbert Gurley, Ph.G.
Brooklyn College of Pharmacy
1927

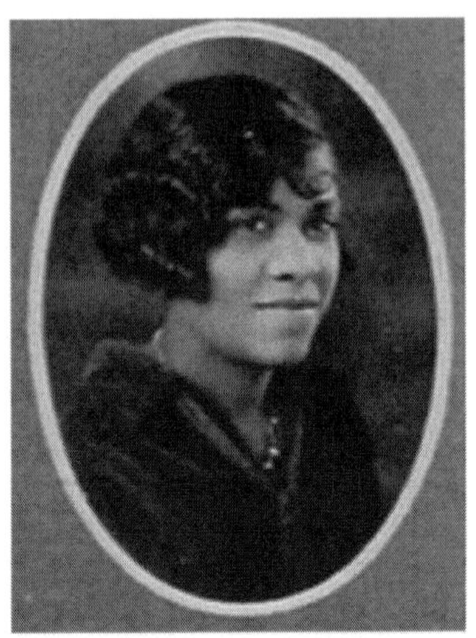

Artelle Levy, Ph.G.
City College of New York
1927

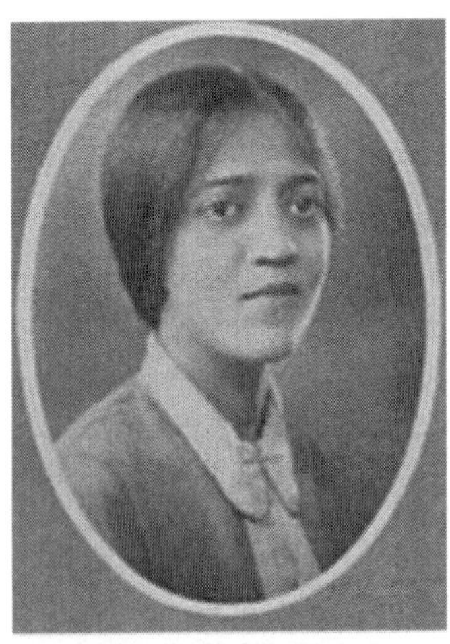

Lillian R. Smith, Ph.G.
City College of New York
1927

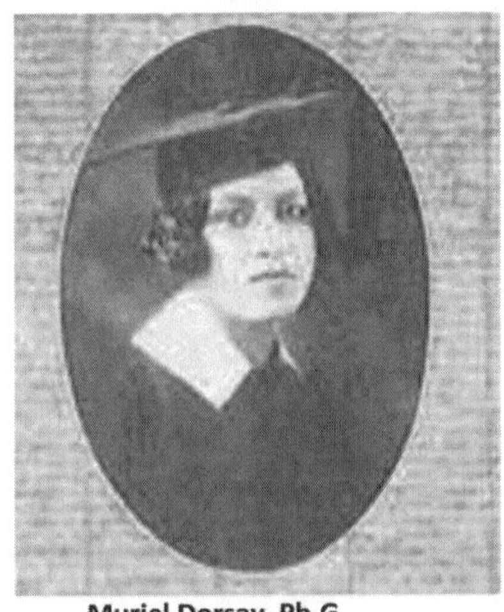

Muriel Dorsay, Ph.G.
College of the City of Detroit
1927

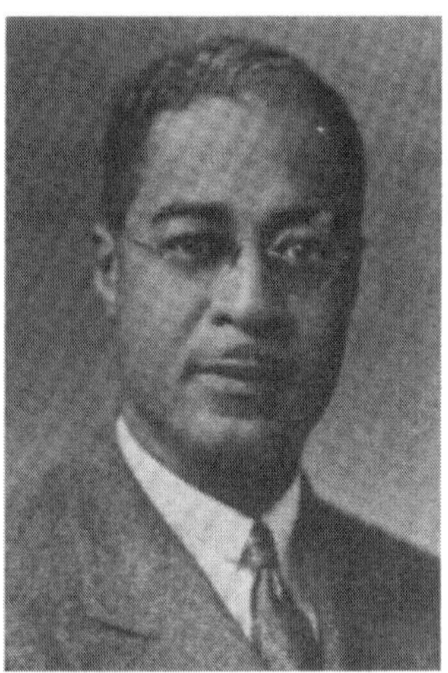

Millard T. Woods, Ph.G. B.S.
University of Nebraska
1928

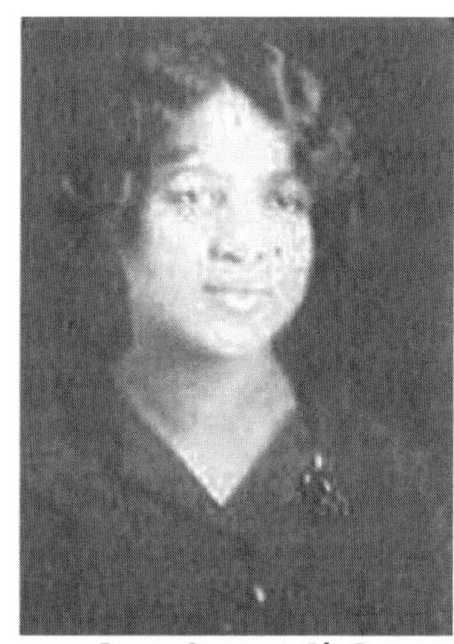

Pansy Stewart, Ph.G.
College of the City of Detroit
1928

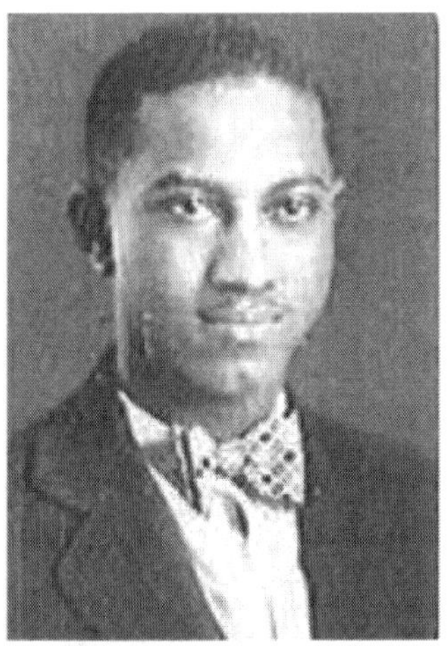

Sidney Barthwell, Ph.G.
College of the City of Detroit
1928

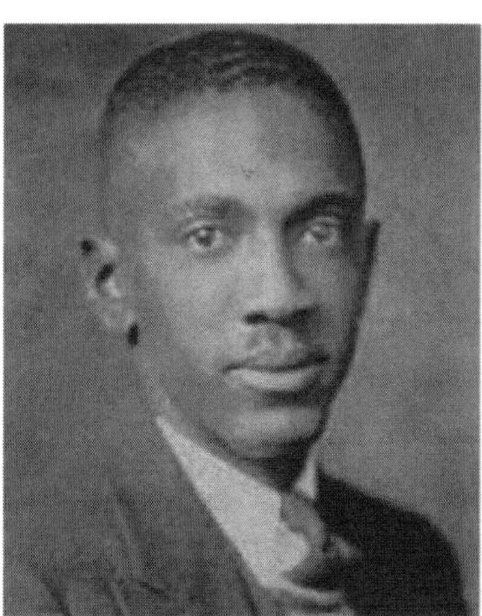

Roscoe G. Henry, Ph.G.
Temple University
1930

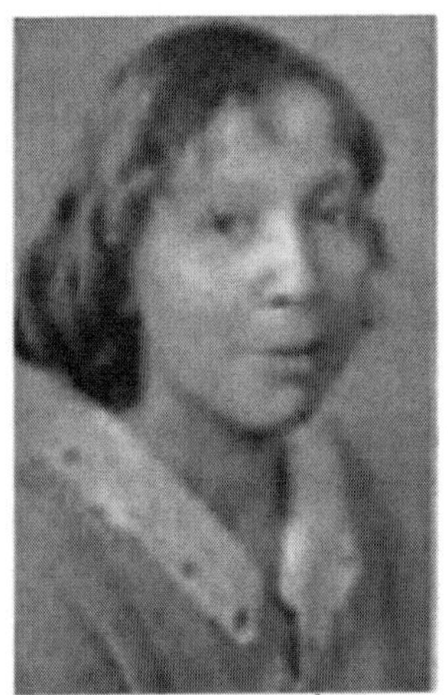
Marie Brown, Ph.G.
University of Iowa
1930

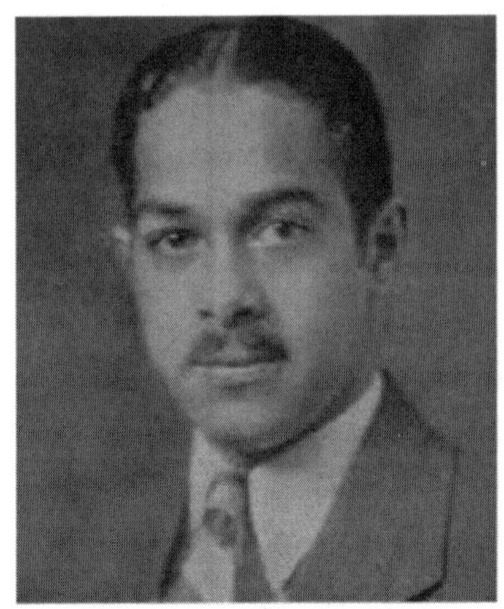
Sylvester H. Johnson, Ph.G.
College of the City of New York
1930

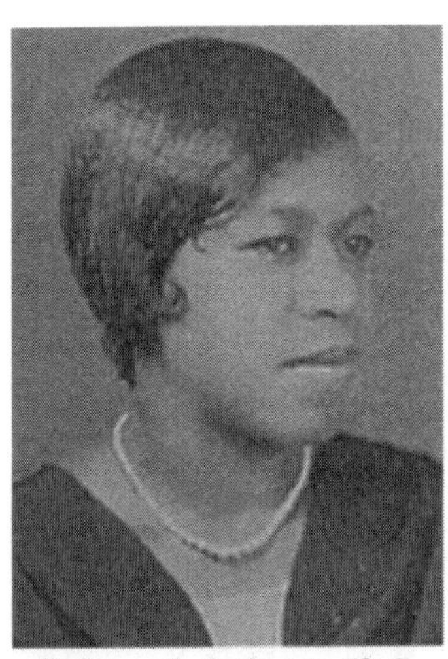
Catharyn O. Anderson, Ph.G.
College of the City of New York
1931

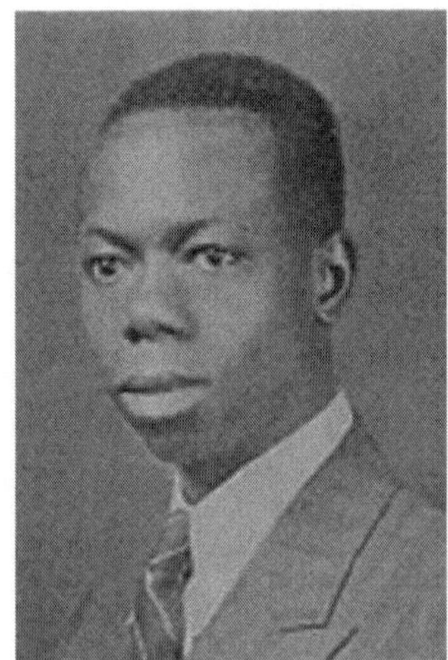
Clifford Albert Williams, Ph.G.
College of the City of New York
1931

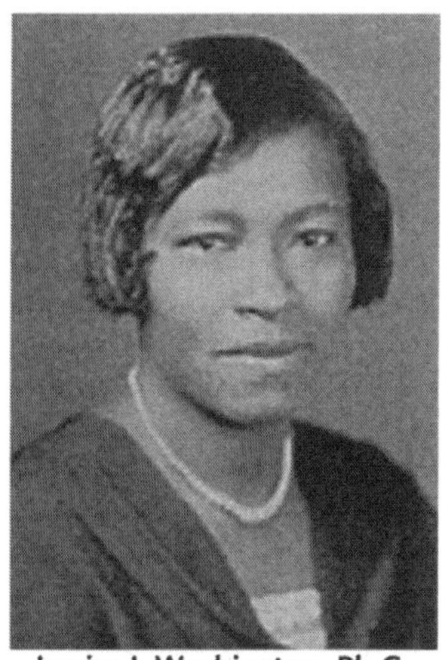

Louise I. Washington, Ph.G.
College of the City of New York
1931

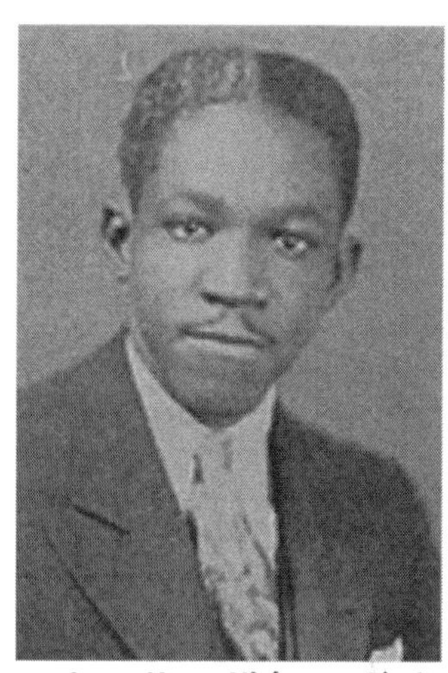

Larry Harry Hickman, Ph.G.
College of the City of New York
1931

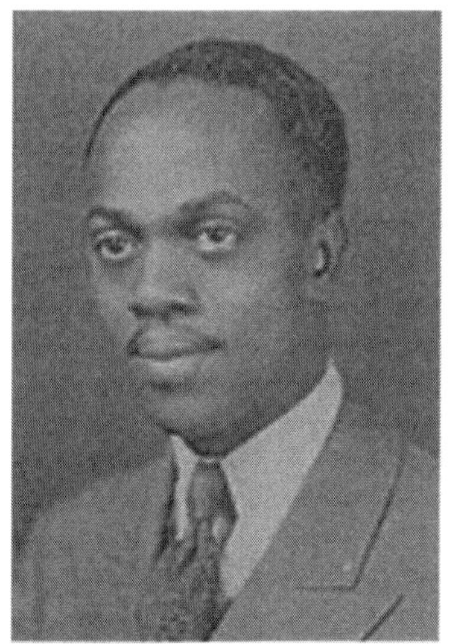

Robert J. Smith, Ph.G.
College of the City of New York
1931

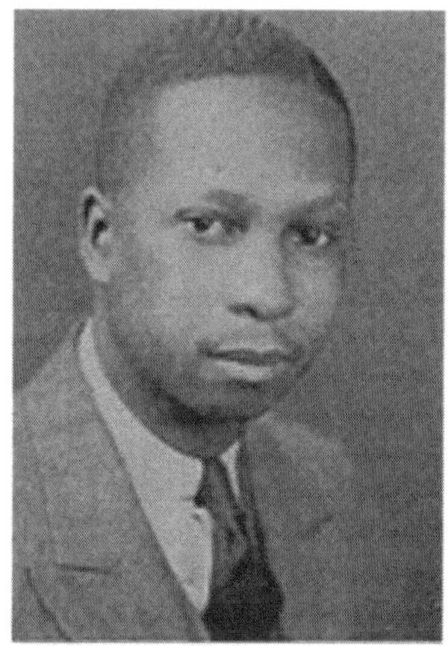

Theodore H. Homer, Ph.G.
College of the City of New York
1931

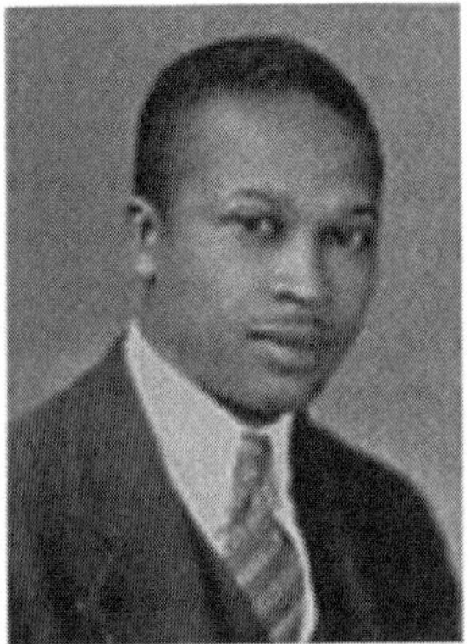

Aubert Evans Reddick, Ph.C.
College of the City of New York
1932

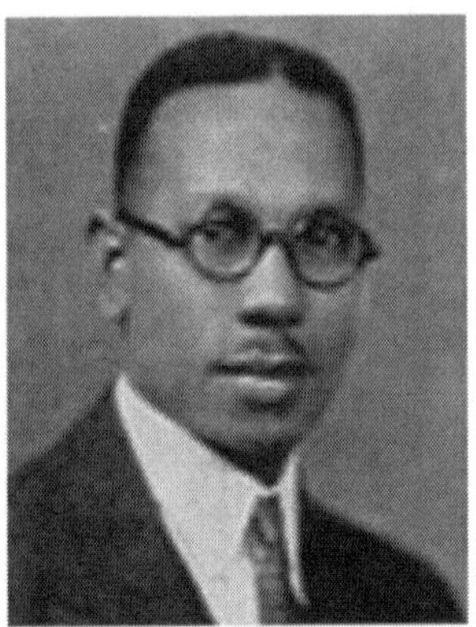

J. Norman Clunie, Ph.C.
College of the City of New York
1932

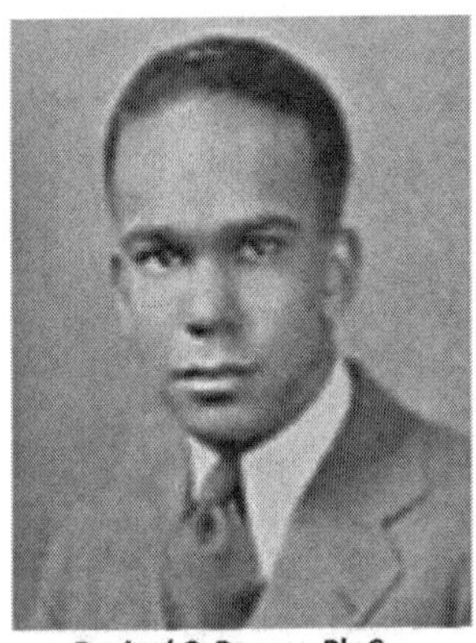

Reginal C. Brown, Ph.C.
College of the City of New York
1932

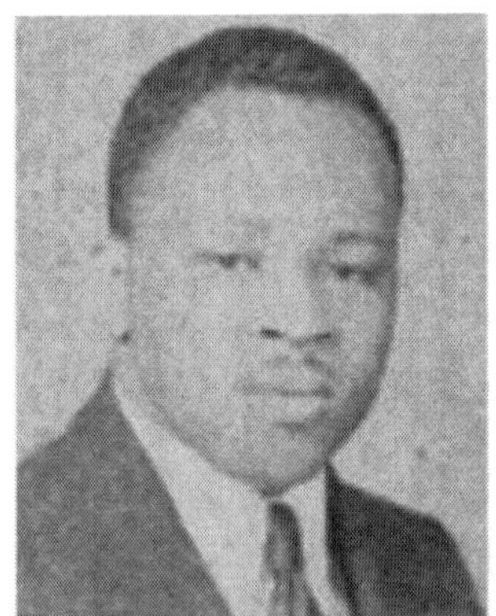

James Bagley
Indianapolis College of Pharmacy
1940

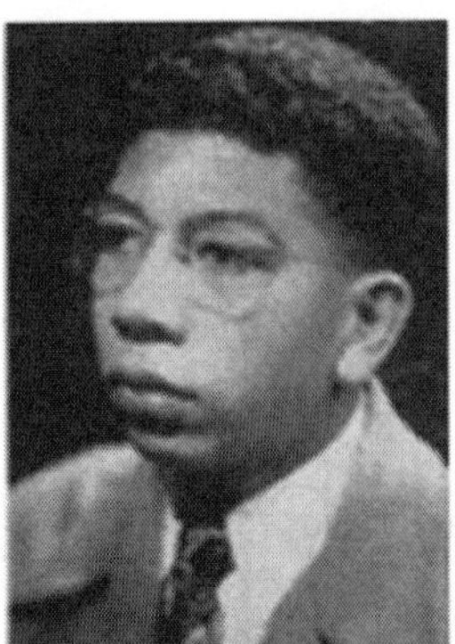

William B. Harrell, Jr., B.S.
University of Washington
1947

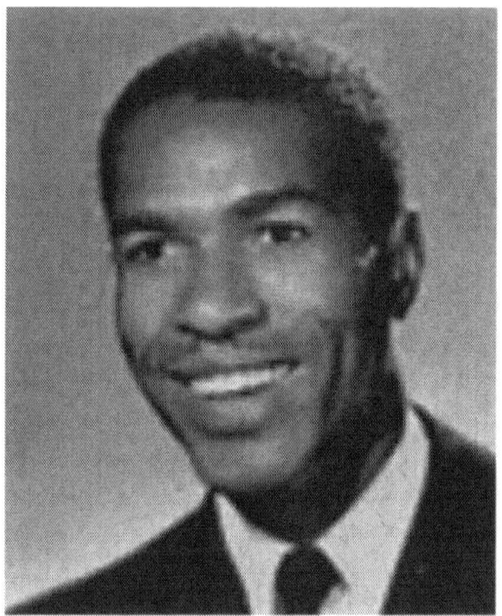

Conrad A. Bohannon, B.S..
University of Arizona
1950

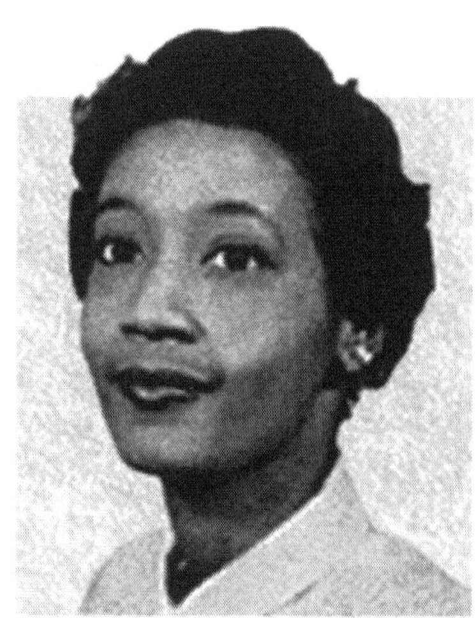

Doris Bryson, B.S.
St. Louis College of Pharmacy
1957

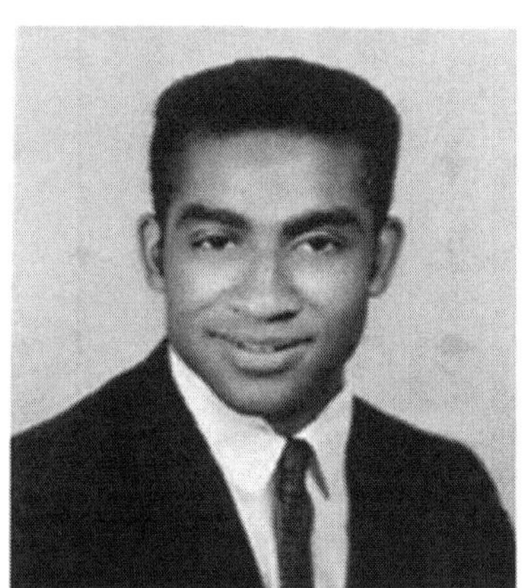

George Mitchell, Jr.
St. Louis College of Pharmacy
1962

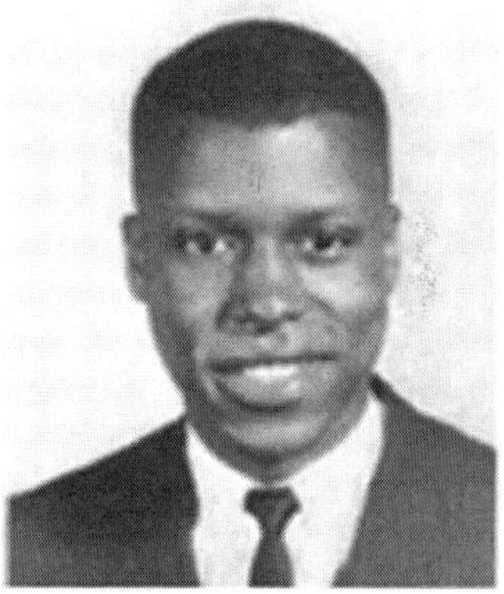

Armon Crawford
St. Louis College of Pharmacy
1963

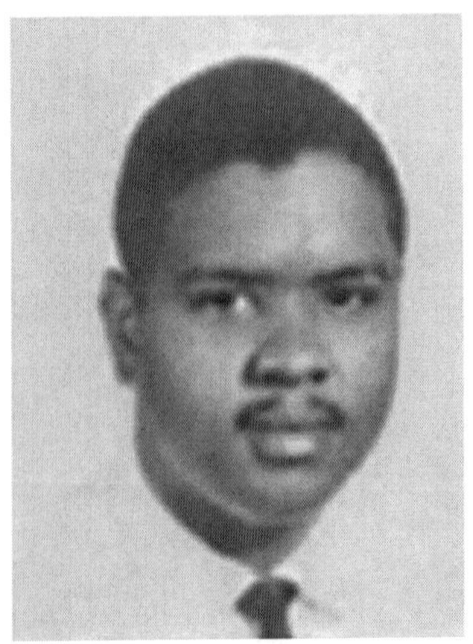

Kenneth Morris
St. Louis College of Pharmacy
1963

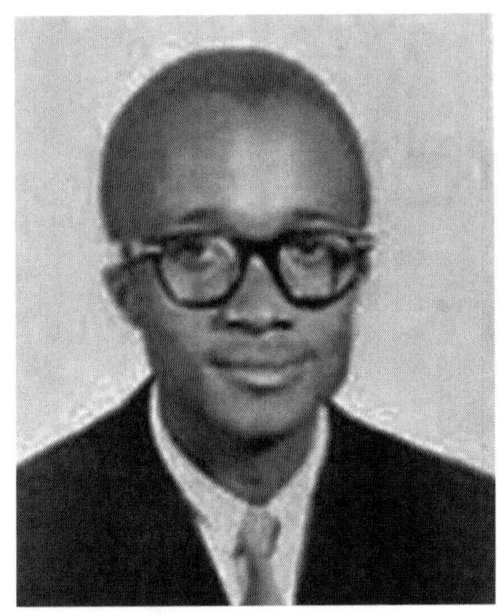

Steve Phillips
St. Louis College of Pharmacy
1963

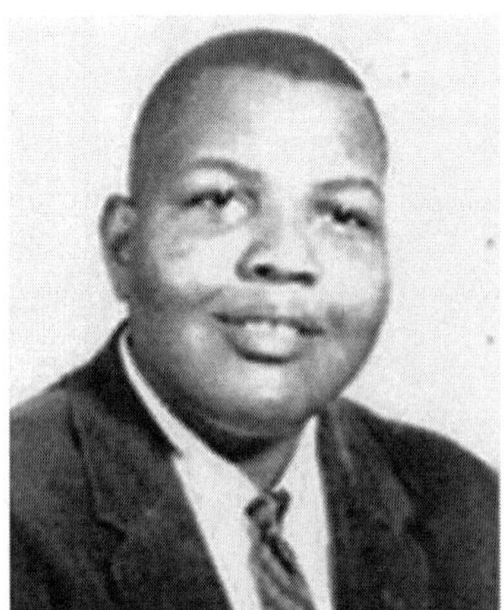

James Tyson
St. Louis College of Pharmacy
1963

Additional Graduates and Students

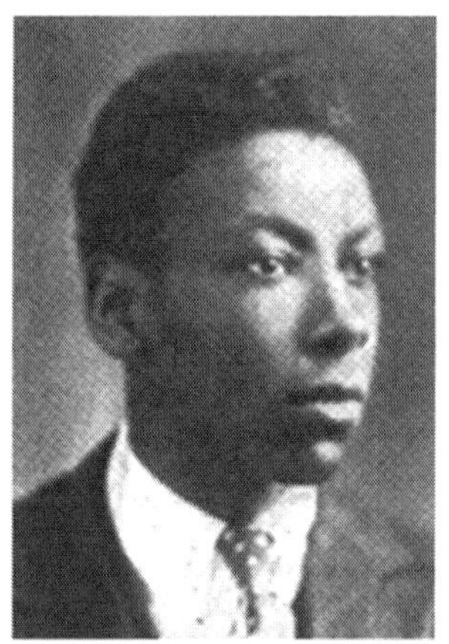

Antoine E. Green, Ph.B.
Massachusetts College of Pharmacy
1921

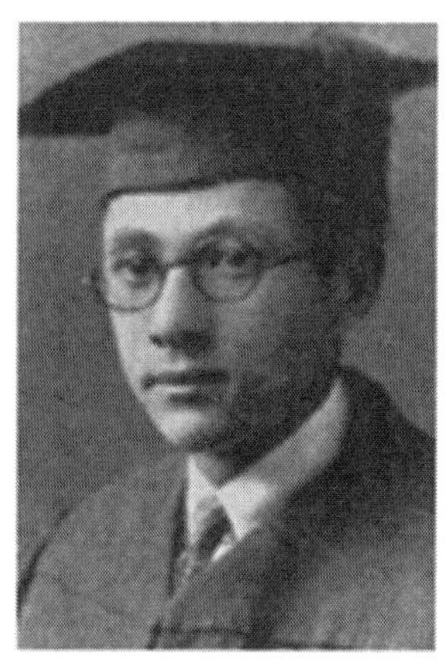

John F. Taylor, Ph.G.
University of Southern California
1924

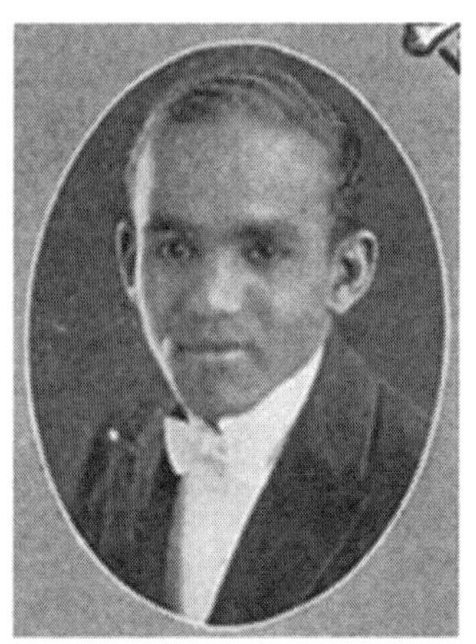

James T. Anderson, Ph.G.
Indianapolis College of Pharmacy
1925

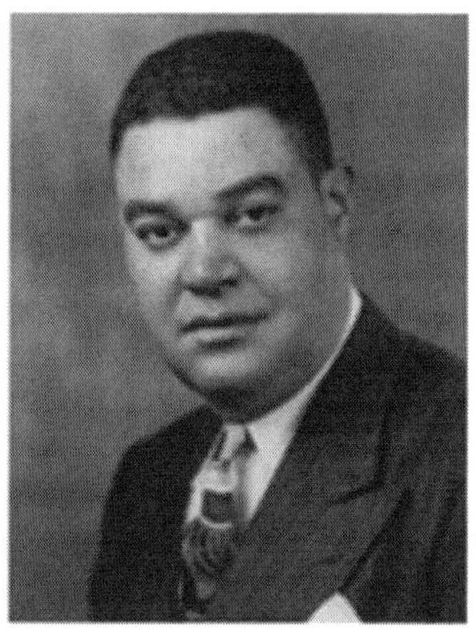

Chauncey I. Cooper, Ph.C.
University of Minnesota
1927

Appendix B
Early African American Pharmacy Graduates and Students from Predominantly White Universities in the South: 1957–1975

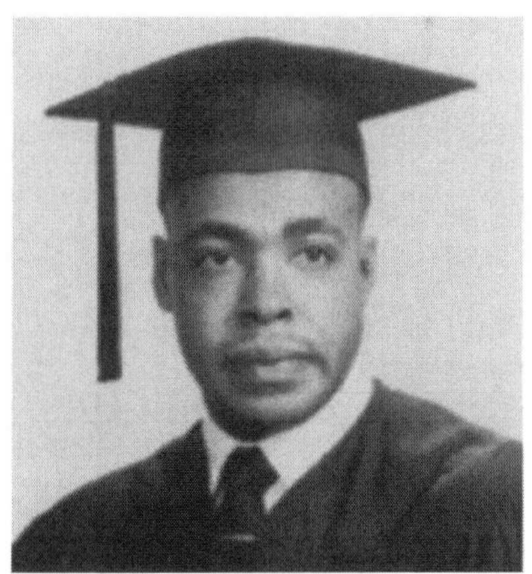

Carl Brooks, B.S.
University of Arkansas
1957

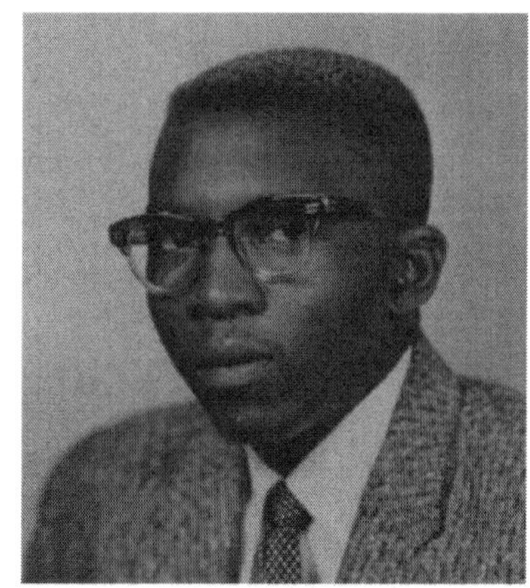

Marion K. Greene
University of Arkansas
1961

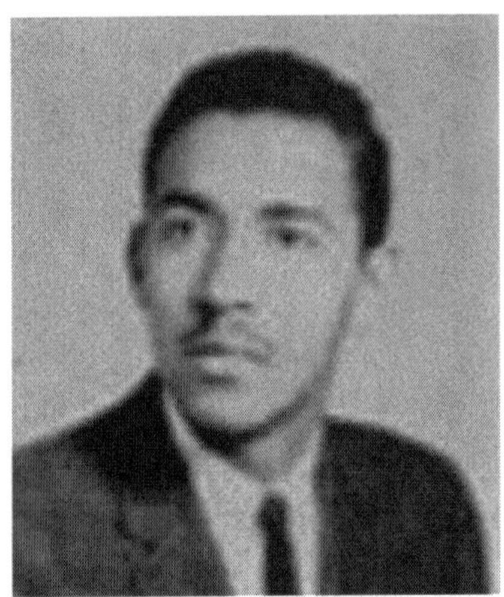

William Wicker, B.S.
University of North Carolina
1965

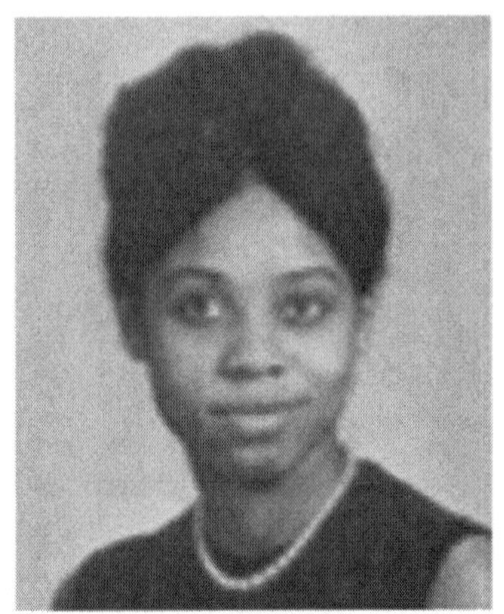

Mona Yvonne Boston, B.S.
University of North Carolina
1967

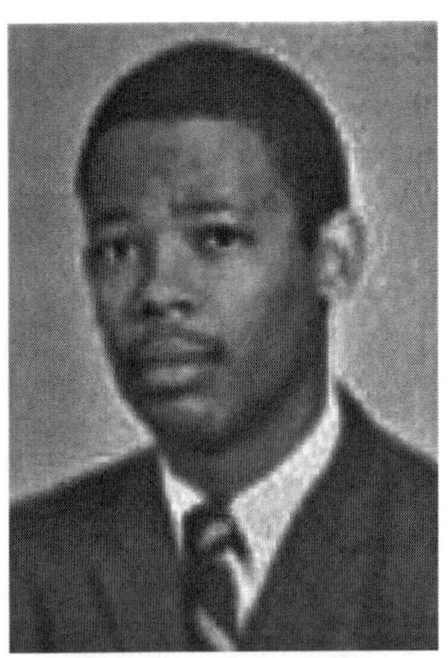

George Leonard, B.S.
University of Mississippi
1969

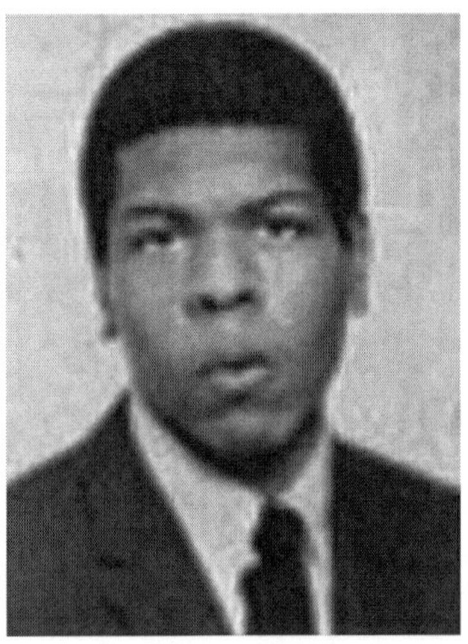

Theron Evans
University of Mississippi
1970

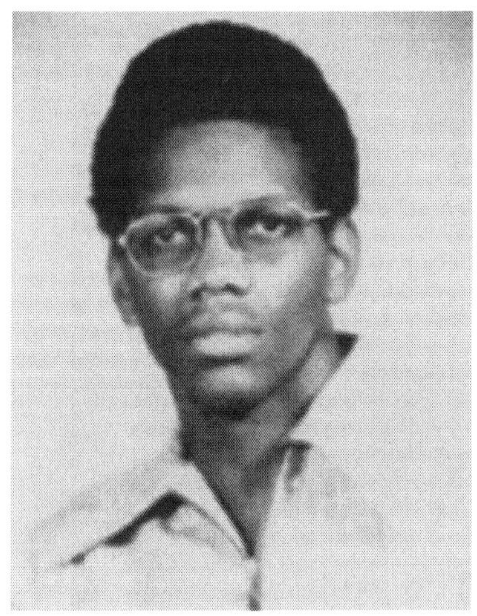

Theotus Butler, B.S.
Samford University
1973

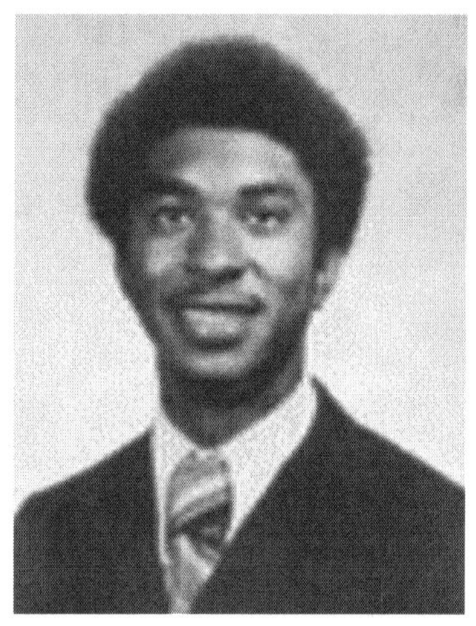

Richard Morgan, B.S.
University of Georgia
1974

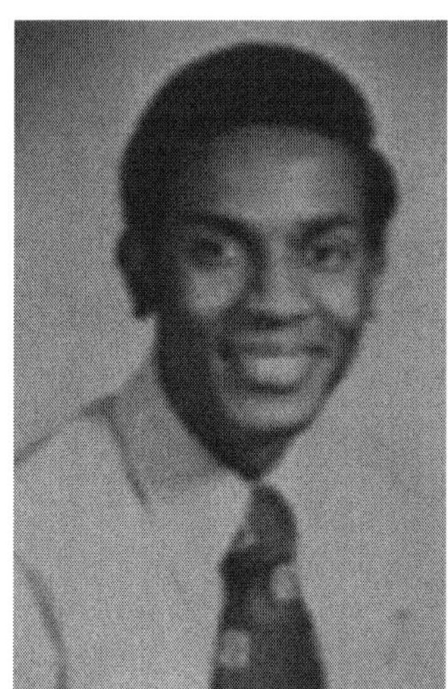

Clarence E. Dubose, B.S.
University of Mississippi
1975

Additional Graduates and Students

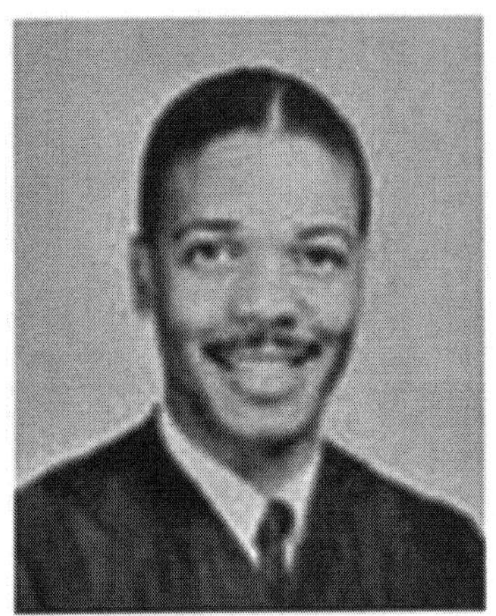

Ronald Myrick, B.S.
Mercer University
1967

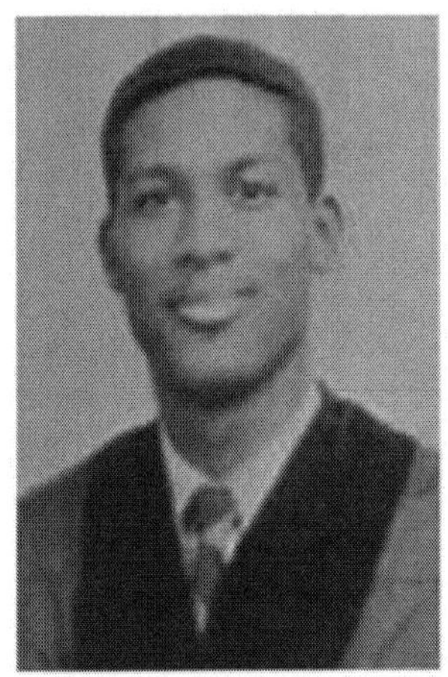

Hewitt Matthews, B.S.
Mercer University
1968

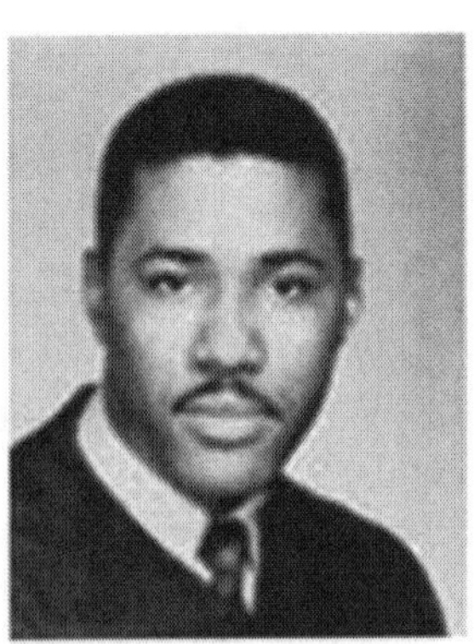

Alphonso Richardson, B.S.
Mercer University
1969

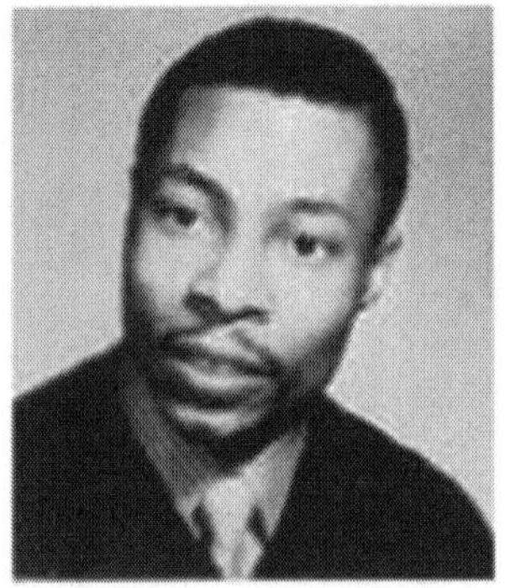

Curtis Smith, B.S.
Mercer University
1969

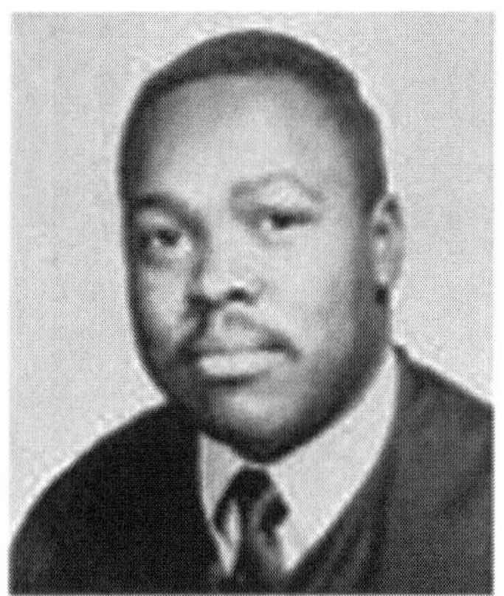

Ronald Briggs, B.S.
Mercer University
1969

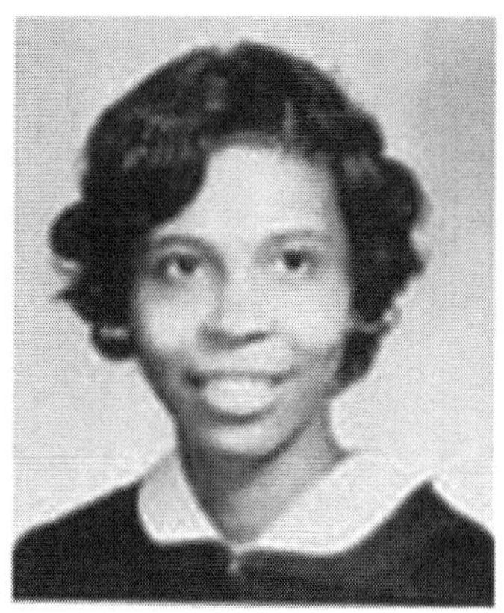

Yvonne Henderson, B.S.
Mercer University
1969

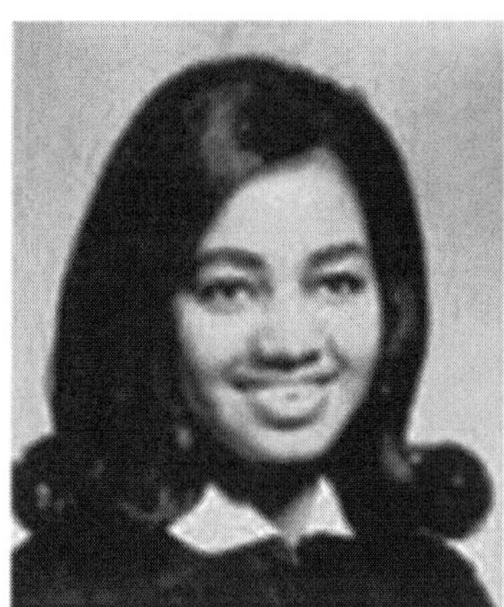

Dorothy Washington, B.S.
Mercer University
1969

Appendix C

Early African American Pharmacy Graduates and Students from Historically Black Colleges and Universities: 1894–1970

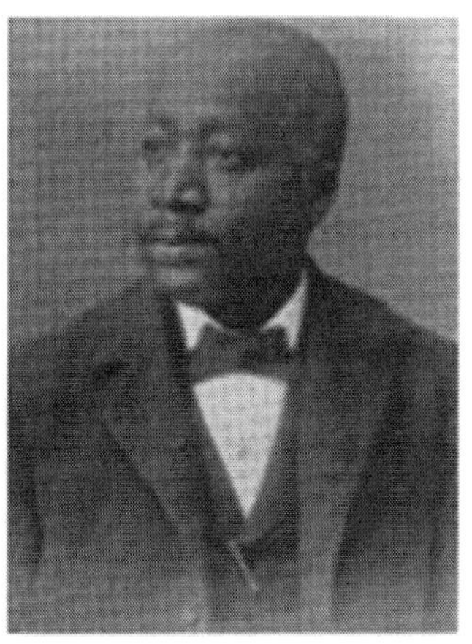

George W. Murray, Phar.D.
Howard University
1894

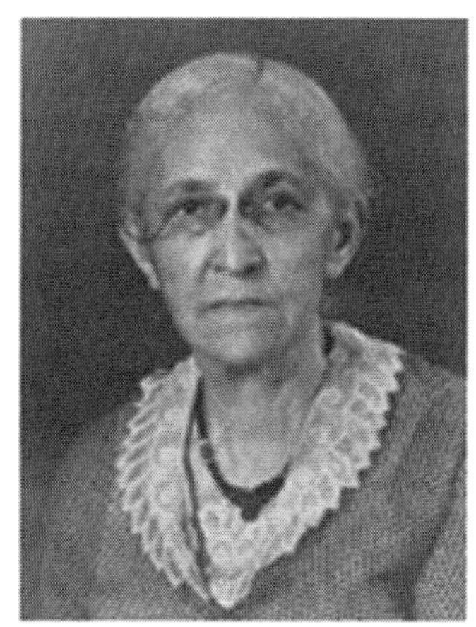

Matilda Lloyd, Ph.G.
Meharry Pharmaceutical College
1894

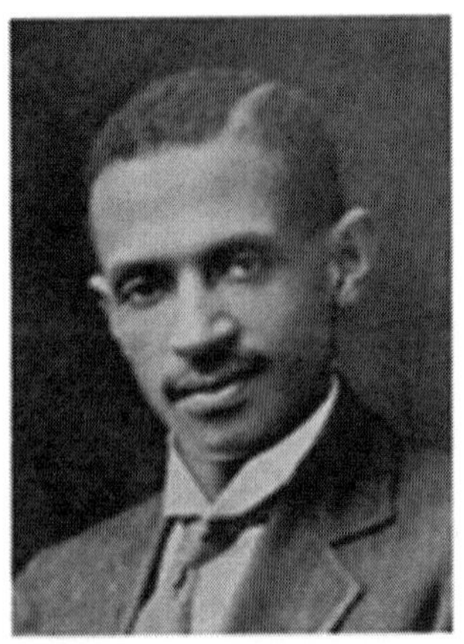

James E Shepard, Ph.G.
Shaw Leonard School of Pharmacy
1894

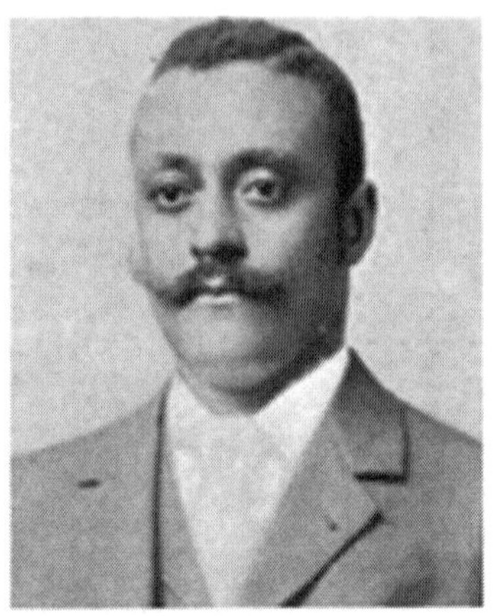

Leroy Henry Harris, Phar.D.
Howard University
1894

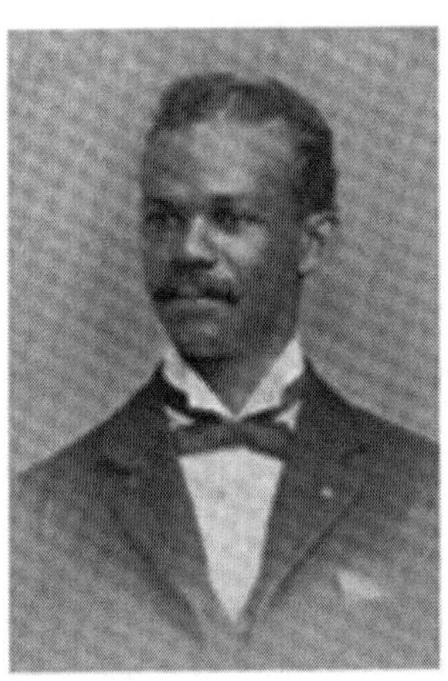

John Oliver Thomas, Phar.D.
Howard University
1895

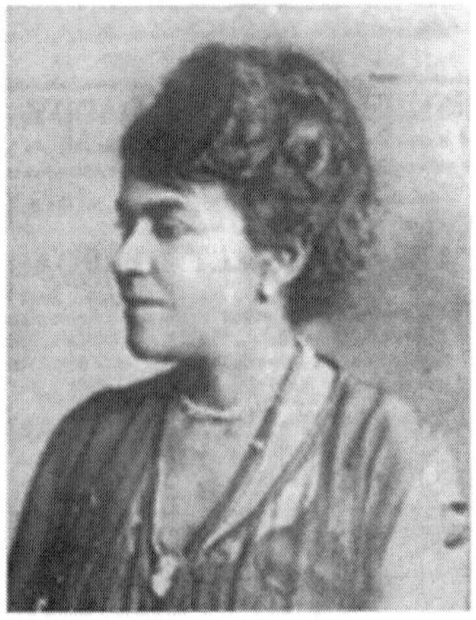

Julia Pearl Hughes, Phar.D.
Howard University
1897

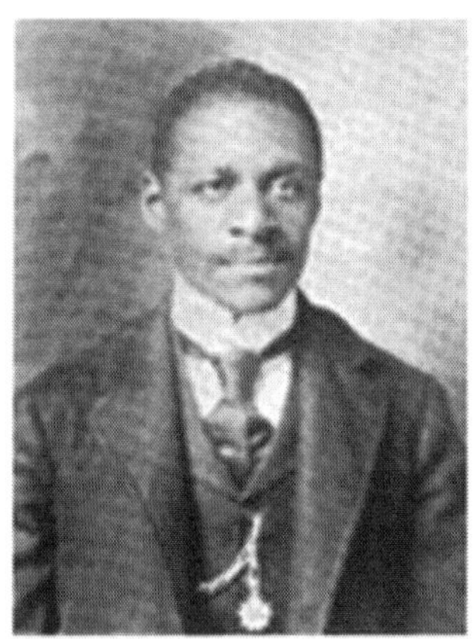

William H. Pipes, Phar.D.
Howard University
1898

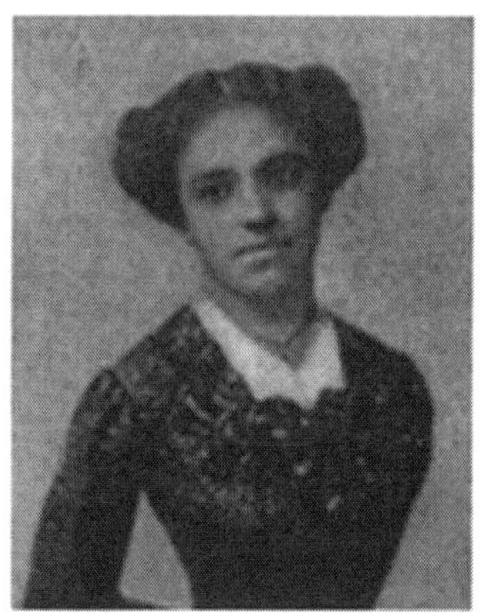

Amanda V. Gray, Phar.D.
Howard University
1903

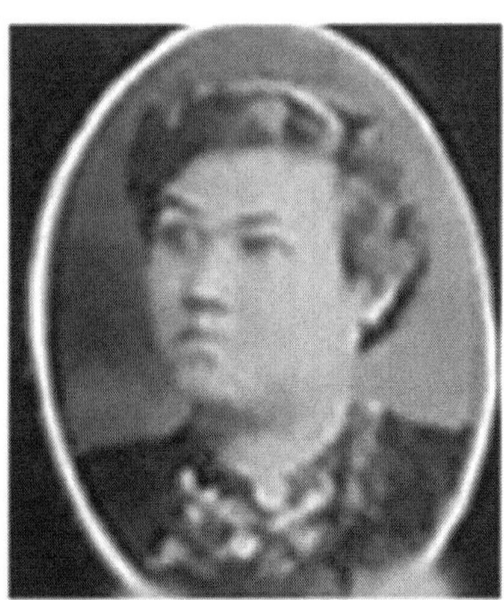

Beebe Stevens Lynk, Ph.C.
University of West Tennessee
1903

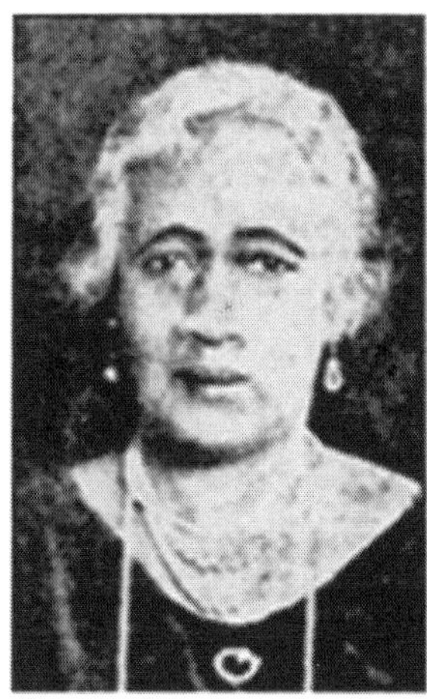

Clara Smyth Taliaferro, Phar.D.
Howard University
1904

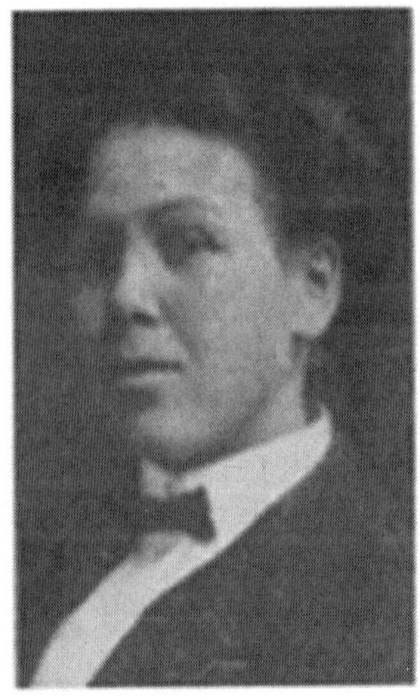

Harriet B. S. Marble, Ph.C.
Meharry Pharmaceutical College
1906

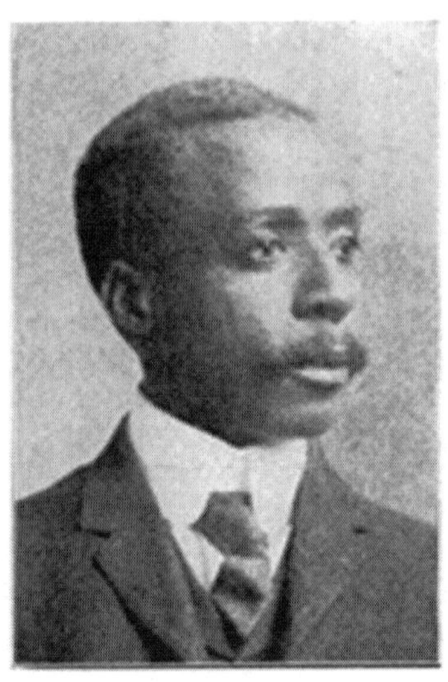

Arthur S. Gray, Phar.D.
Howard University
1910

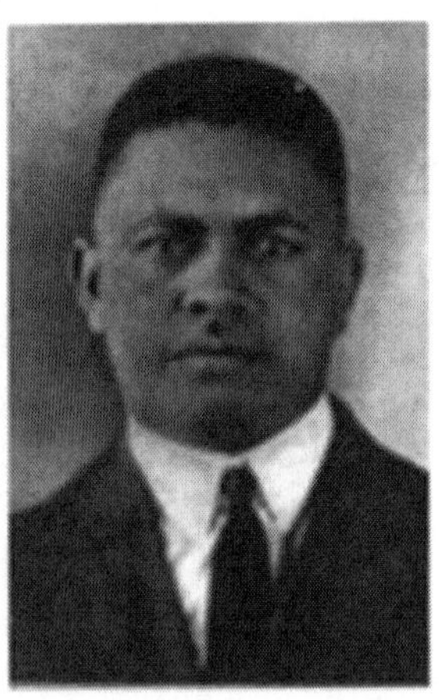

Robert McCants Harris, Ph.C.
Shaw Leonard School of Pharmacy
1914

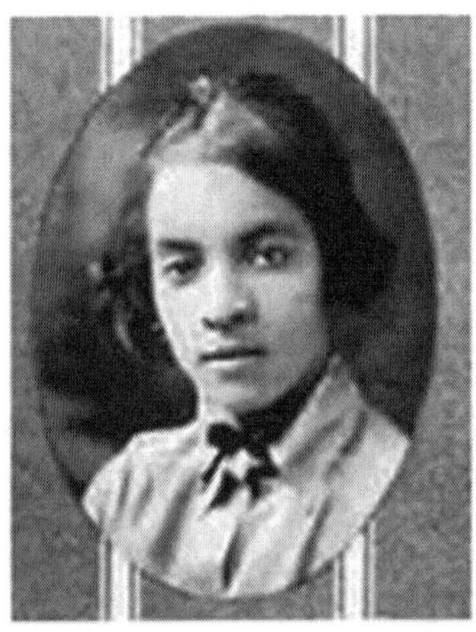

Antoinette J. Sampson, Ph.C.
Howard University
1921

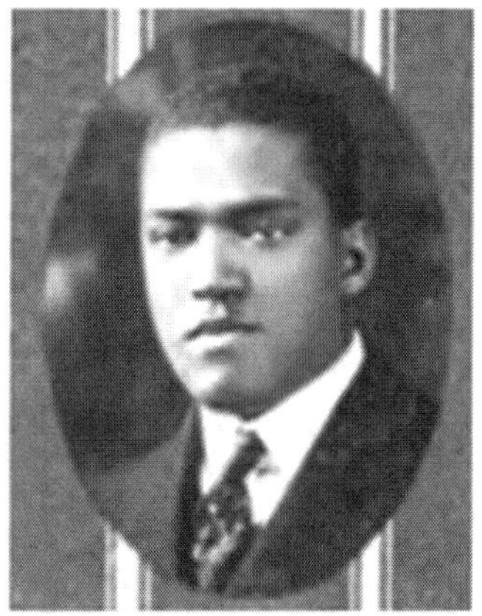

Clarence A. Carter, Ph.C.
Howard University
1921

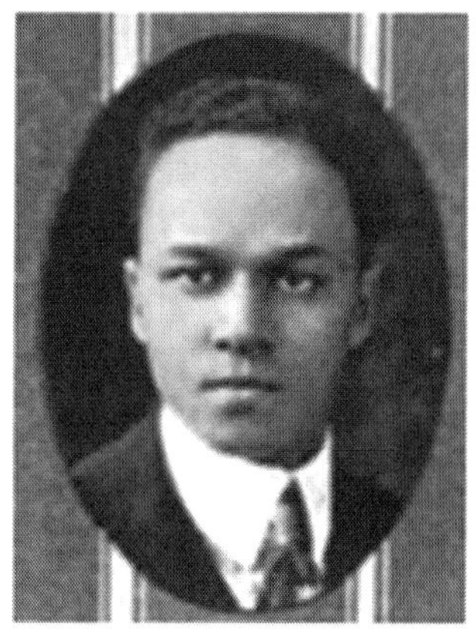

Clay R. Beckley, Ph.C.
Howard University
1921

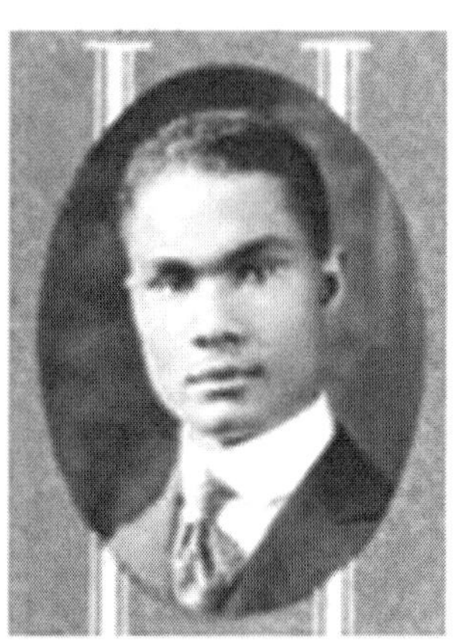

Edward A. Vallate, Ph.C.
Howard University
1921

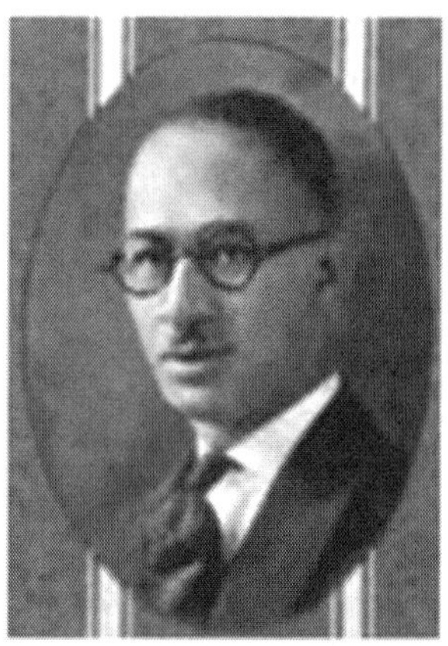

Jesse E. Dickson, Ph.C.
Howard University
1921

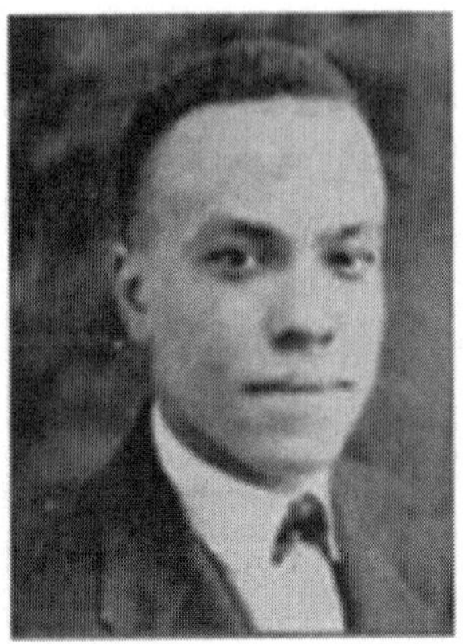

Albert Corum, Phar.D.
Howard University
1922

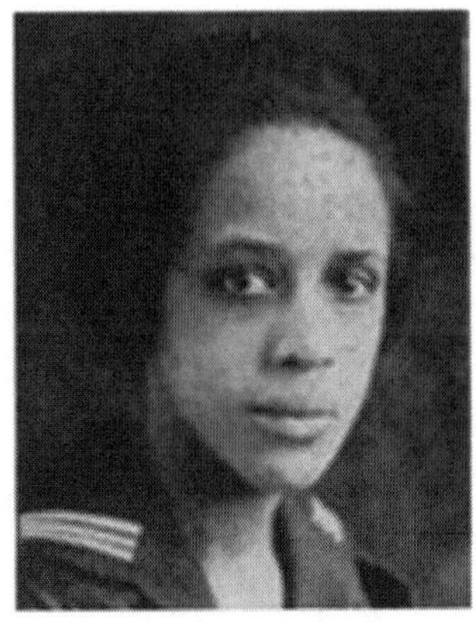

Katy E. Gee, Phar.D.
Howard University
1922

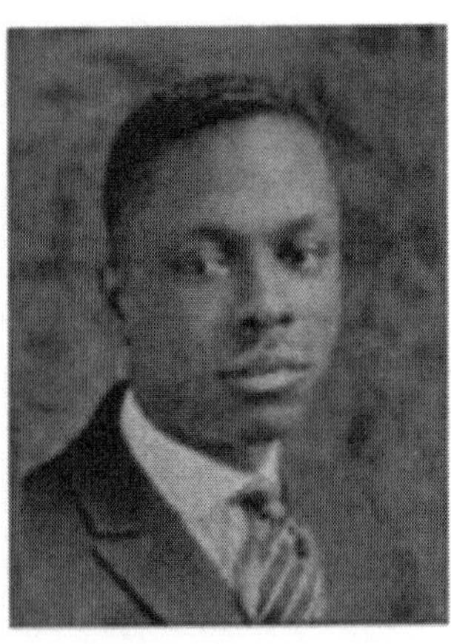

Creed W. Parker, Phar.D.
Howard University
1922

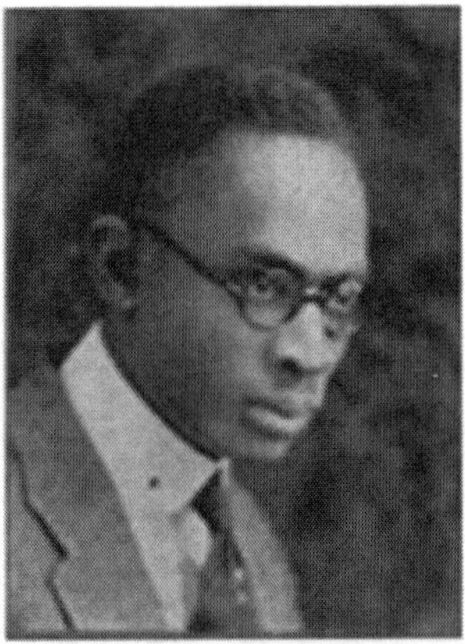

Lorraine E. Jones, Phar.D.
Howard University
1922

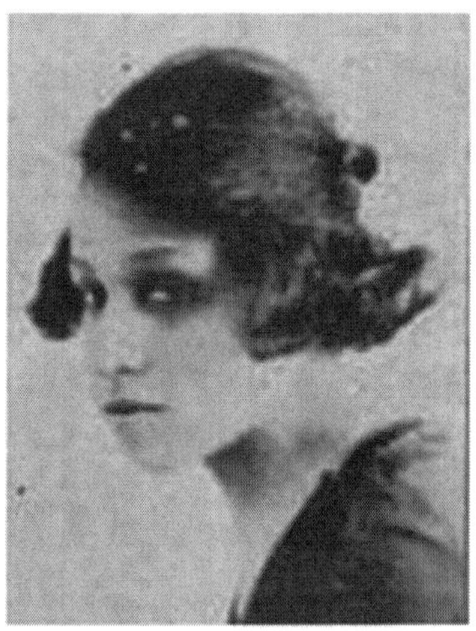

Lillian R. Skinker, Phar.D.
Howard University
1922

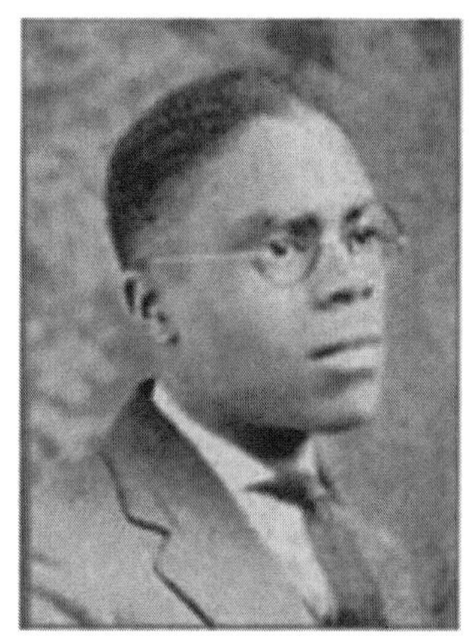

Luzerne W. Costen, Phar.D.
Howard University
1922

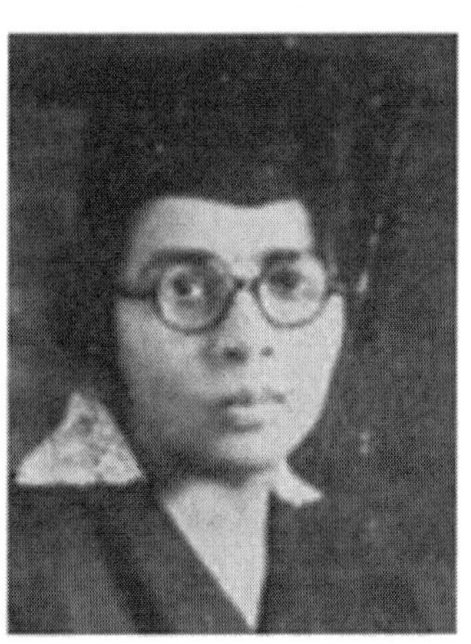

Lillian R. Woodyard, Phar.D.
Howard University
1922

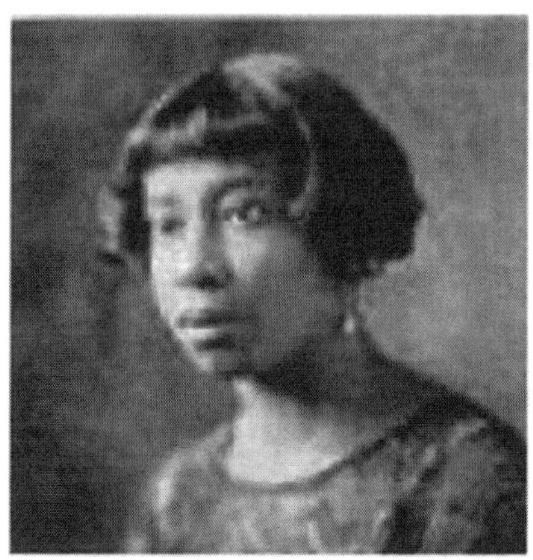

Jennie K. Pusey, Phar.D.
Howard University
1925

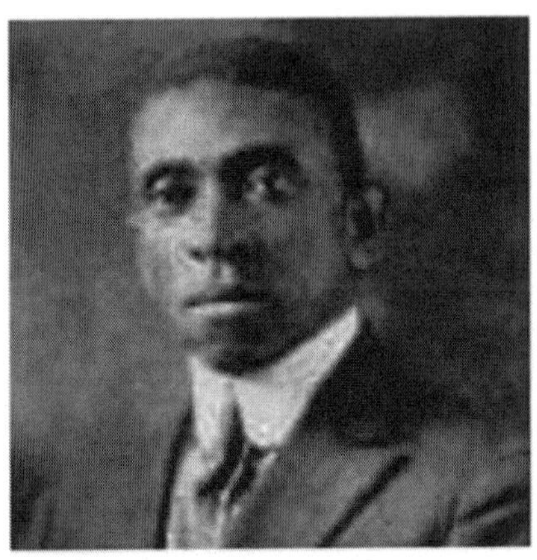

Clarence E. Austin, Phar.D.
Howard University
1925

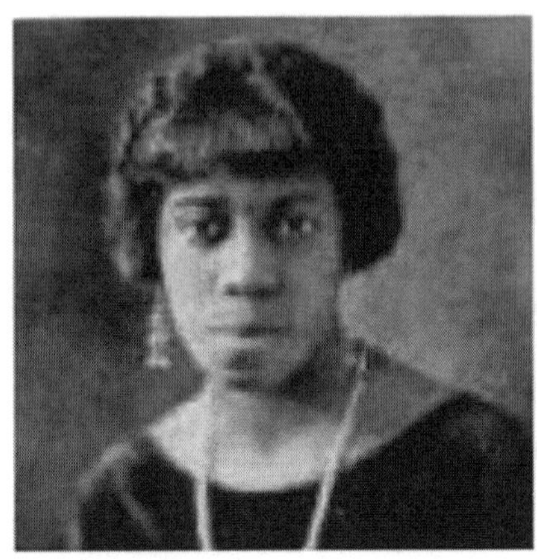

Mozella E. Lewis, Phar.D.
Howard University
1925

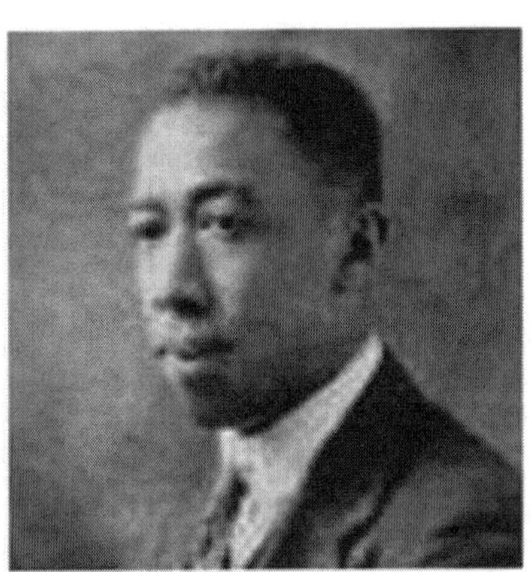

Daniel W. Portlock, Phar.D.
Howard University
1925

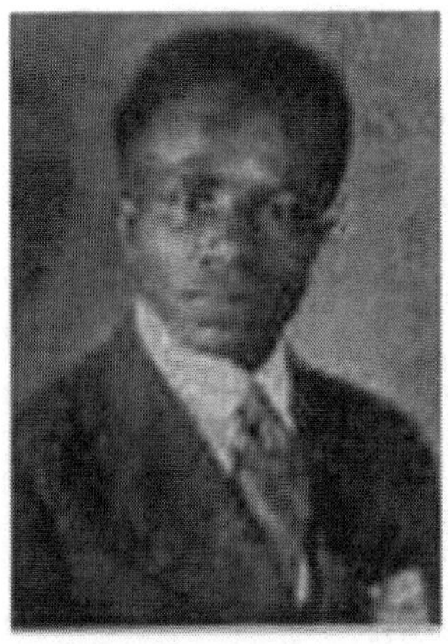

Henry C. Eccles, Phar.D.
Howard University
1926

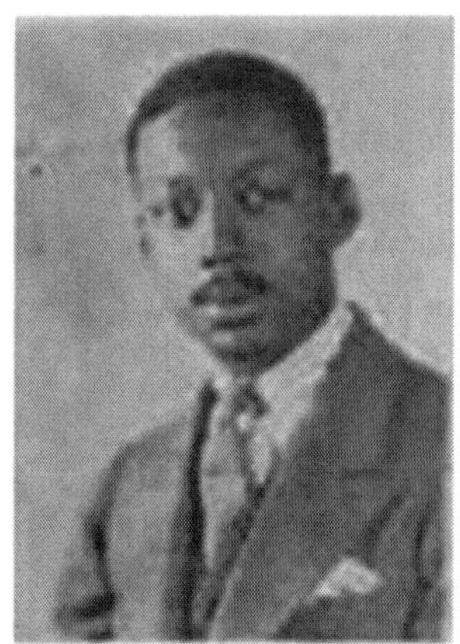

Frank B. Mantley, Phar.D.
Howard University
1926

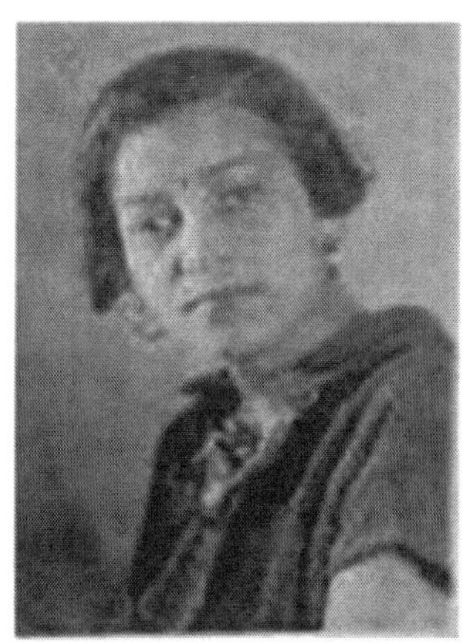

Alice L. A. Tompkins, Phar.D.
Howard University
1926

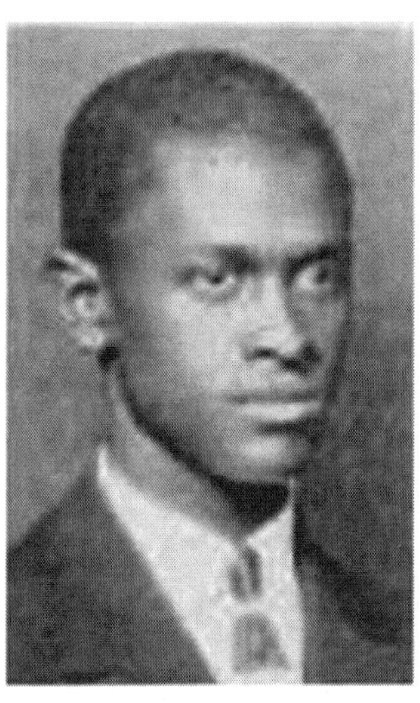

George L. Samuels, Phar.D.
Howard University
1927

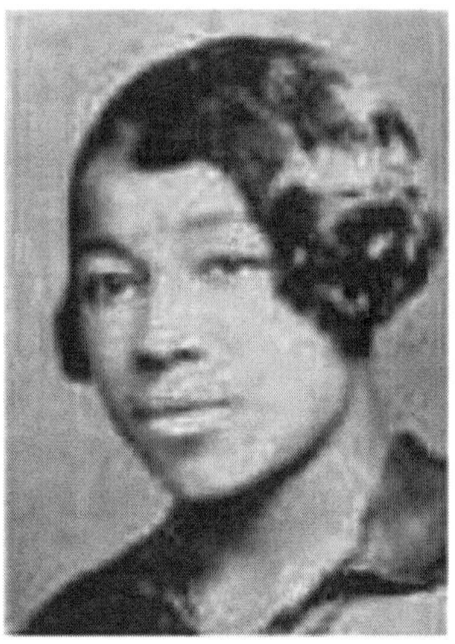

Leona R. McCants, Phar.D.
Howard University
1927

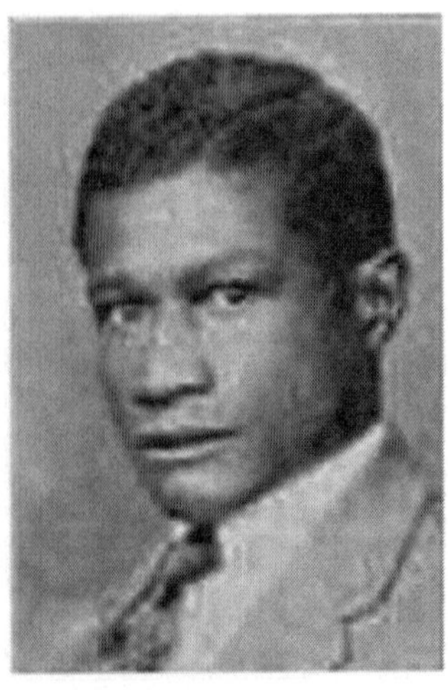

Richard A. King, Phar.D.
Howard University
1927

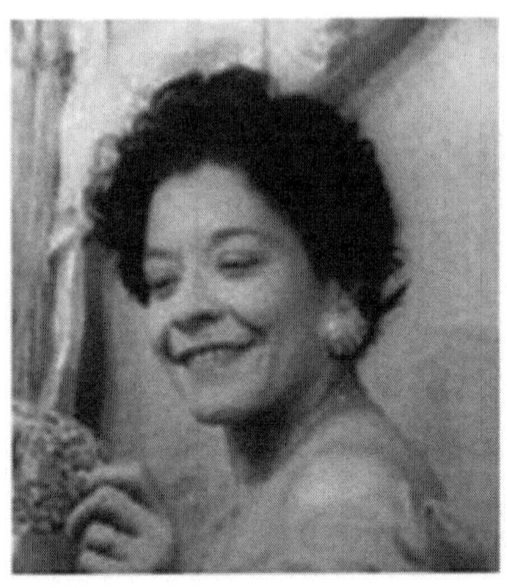

Mollie V. Lewis (Moon) Ph.C.
Meharry Pharmaceutical College
1928

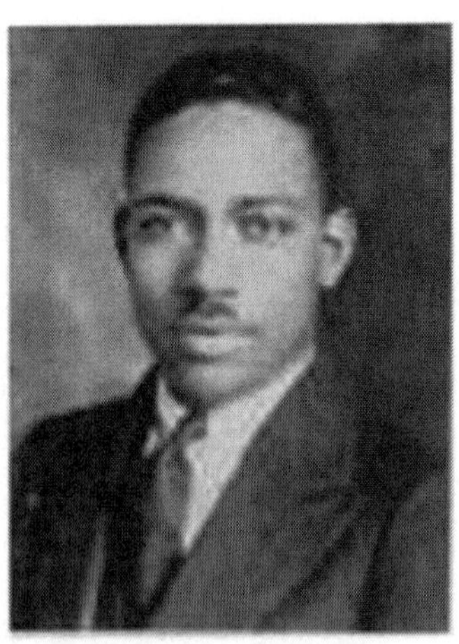

John A. Martin, Phar.D.
Howard University
1929

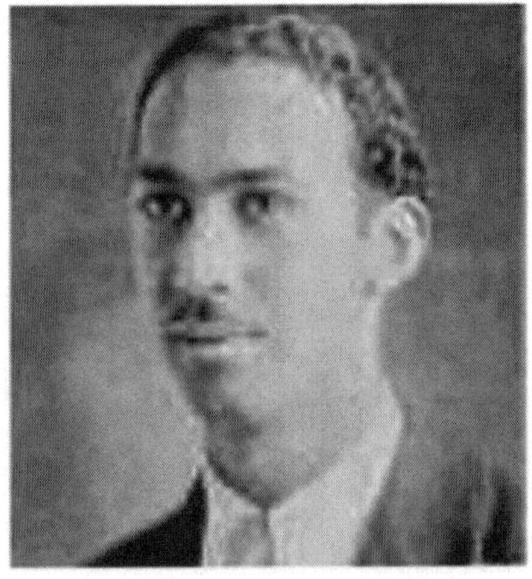

Claude E. Anderson, Phar.D.
Howard University
1929

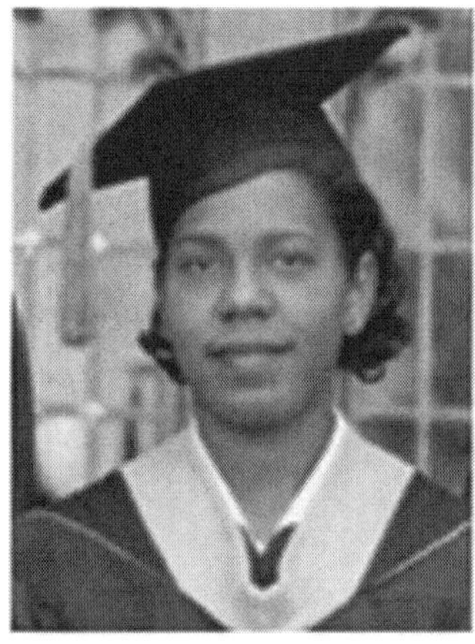

Thelma R. Cunningham, B.S.
Xavier University
1938

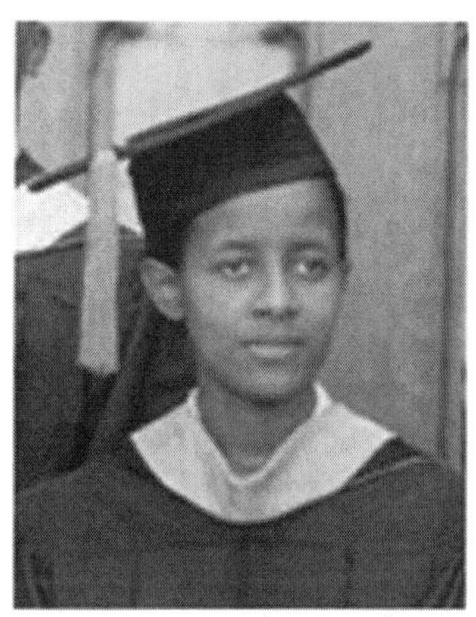

Pearl Inez Barnes, B.S.
Xavier University
1938

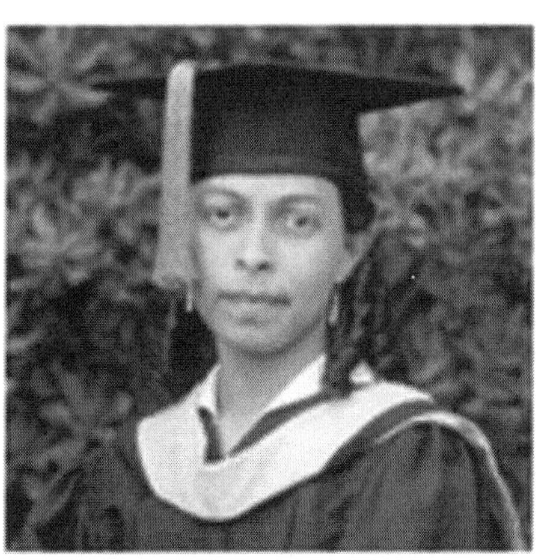

Ethel M. Trudeau, B.S.
Xavier University
1940

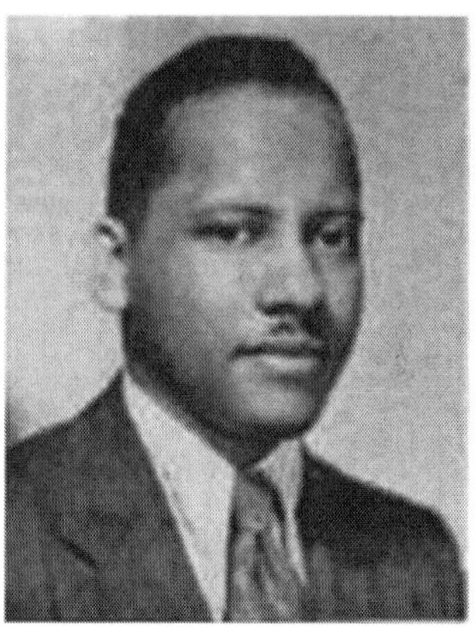

Frank O. Colbert, B.S.
Howard University
1943

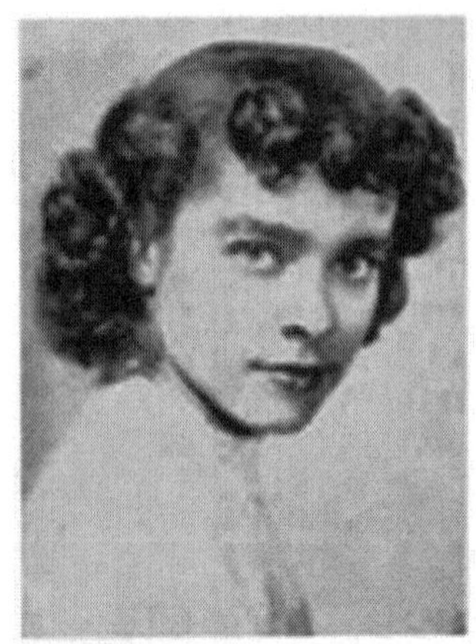

Mary E. Wingate, B.S.
Howard University
1943

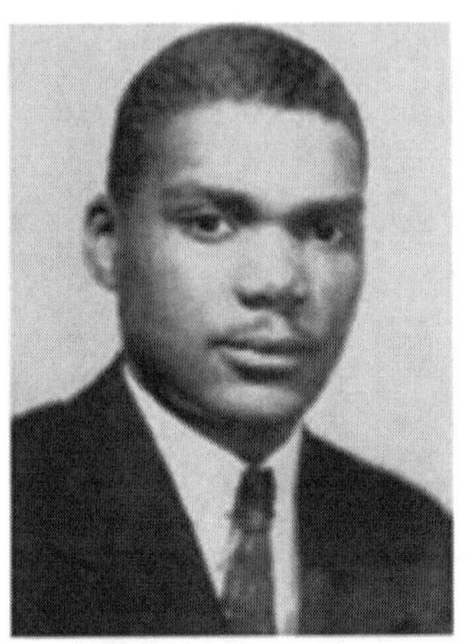

Robert A. Crump, B.S.
Howard University
1943

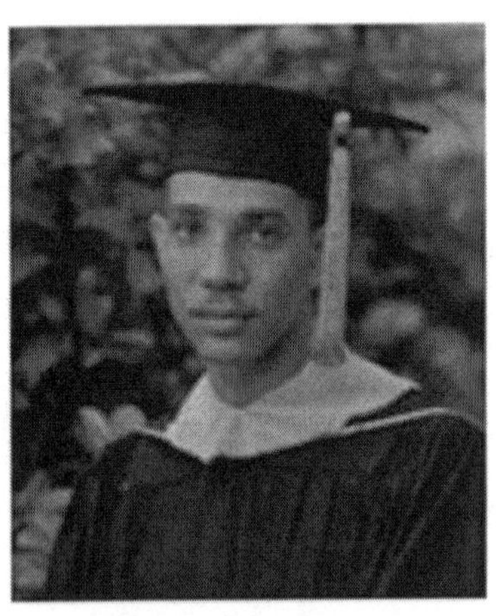

Gilbert Rochon, B.S.
Xavier University
1945

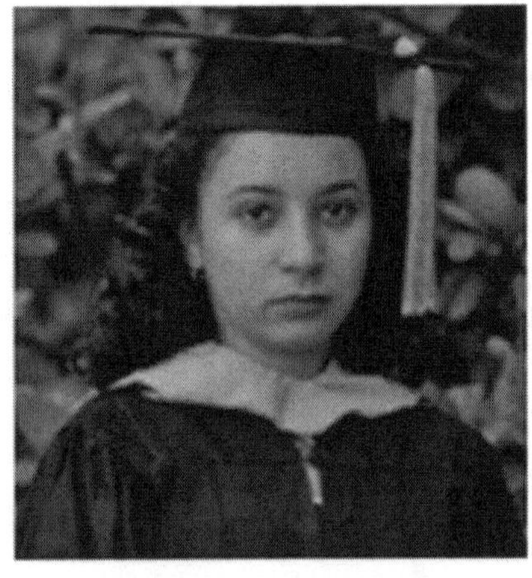

Rose Marie Walker, B.S.
Xavier University
1944

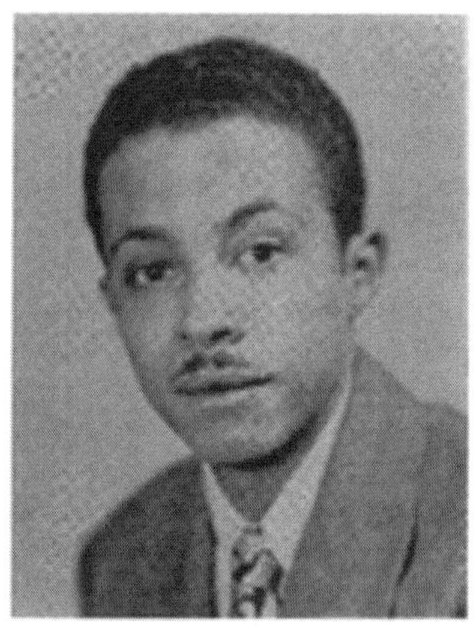

Clement M. Neely, B.S.
Howard University
1946

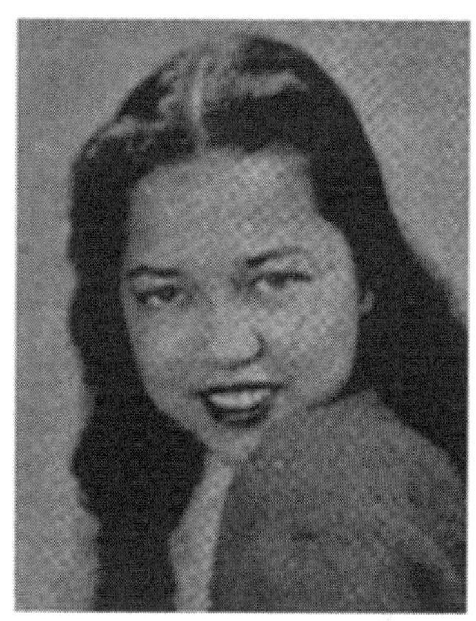

Flora Maria Tann, B.S.
Howard University
1946

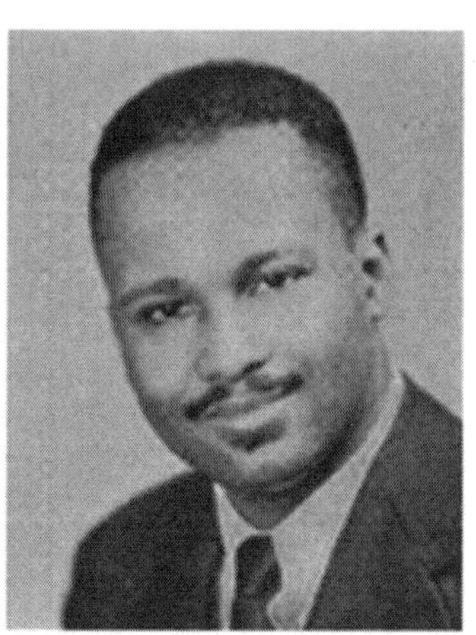

Joseph W. Butcher, B.S.
Howard University
1946

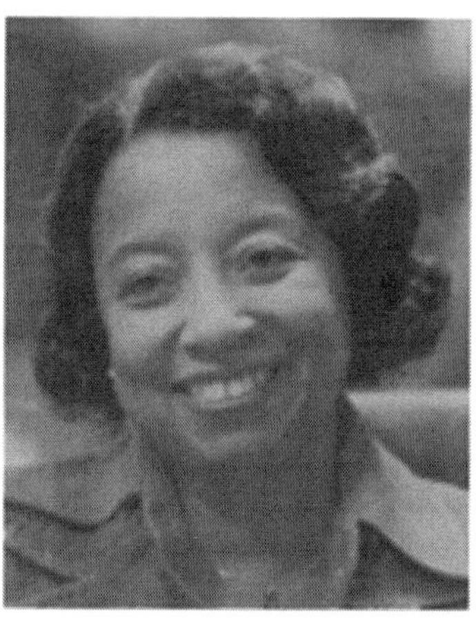

Mary Munson Runge, B.S.
Xavier University
1948

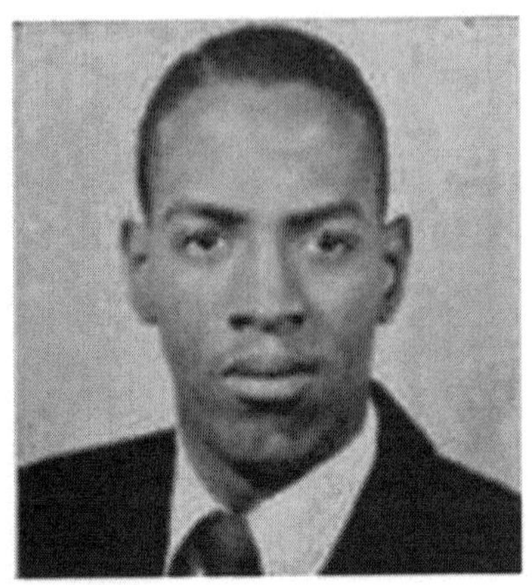

Clarence E. Beverly, B.S.
Howard University
1949

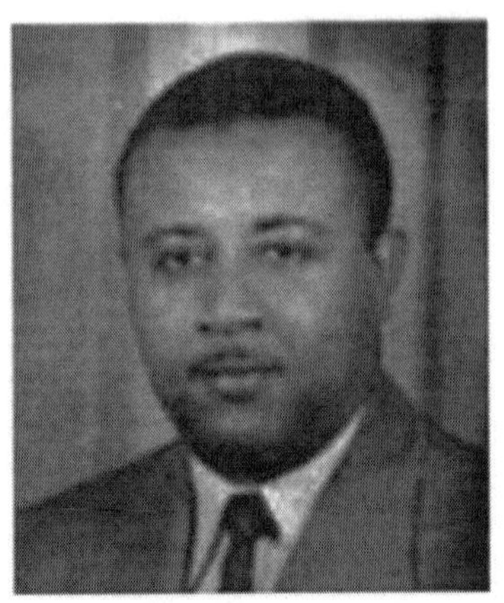

Leo R. Trotter, B.S.
Howard University
1949

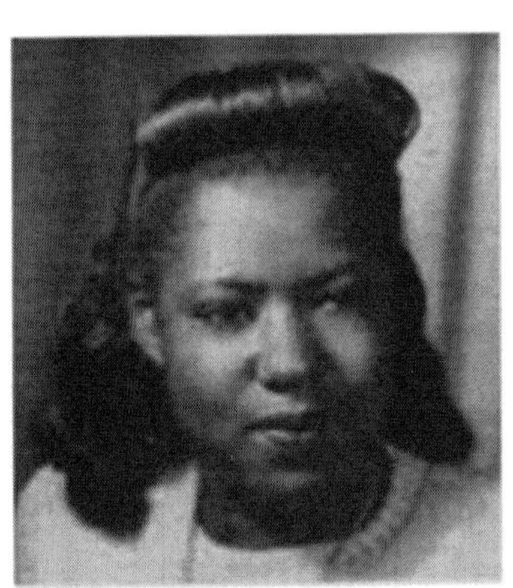

Ruth E. Smith, B.S.
Howard University
1949

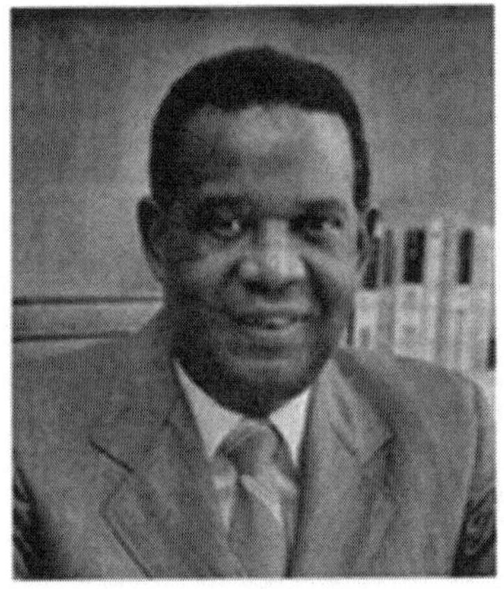

Aaron E. Henry, B.S.
Xavier University
1950

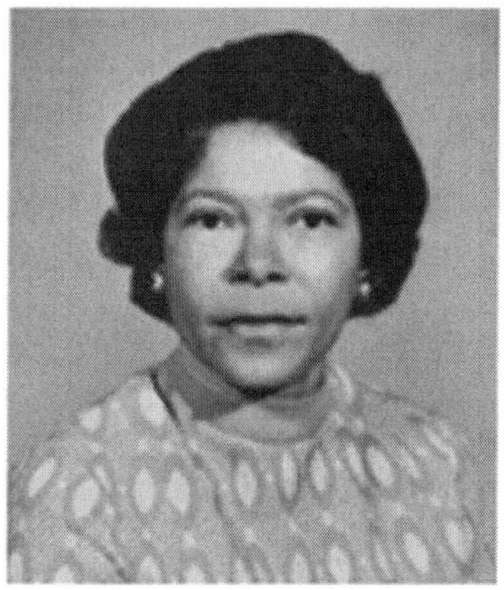

Dolores Cooper Shockley, B.S.
Xavier University
1951

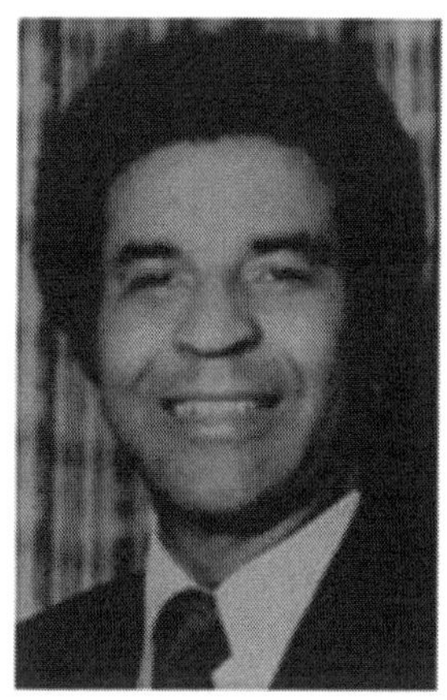

Alvin J. Boutte, B.S.
Xavier University
1951

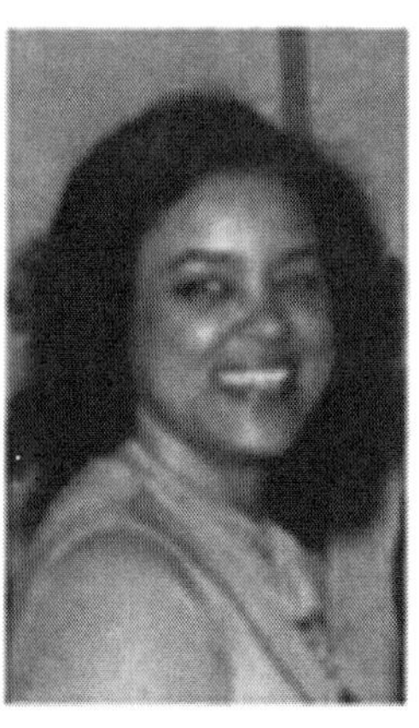

Marie L. Best, B.S.
Xavier University
1951

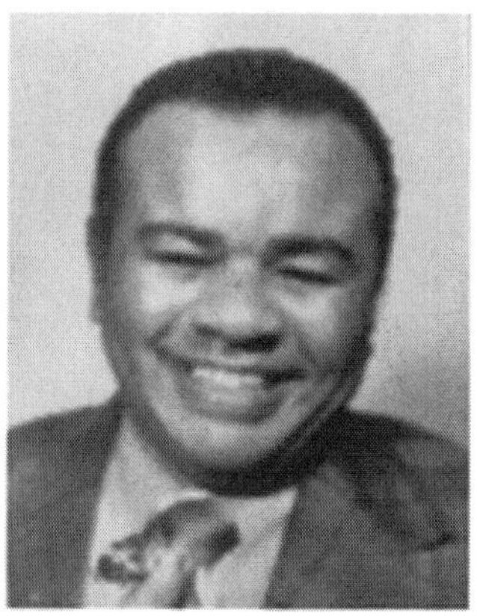

Eugene Hickman, Sr., B.S.
Texas Southern University
1952

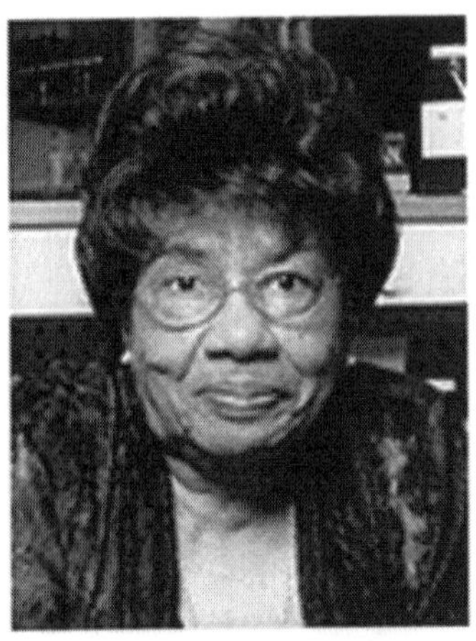

Geraldine Roberts, B.S.
Florida A&M University
1954

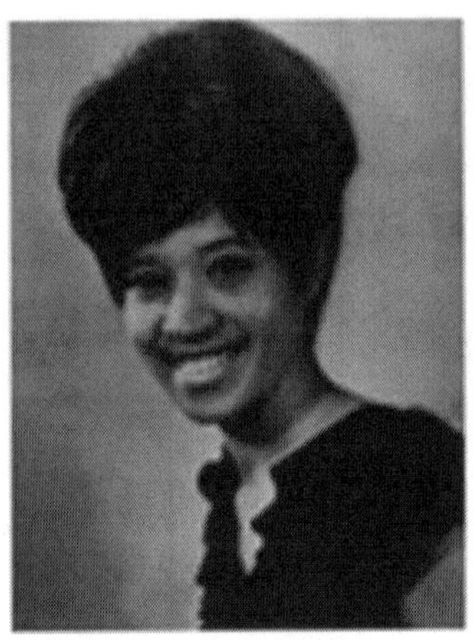

Regina Jollivette, B.S.
Howard University
1965

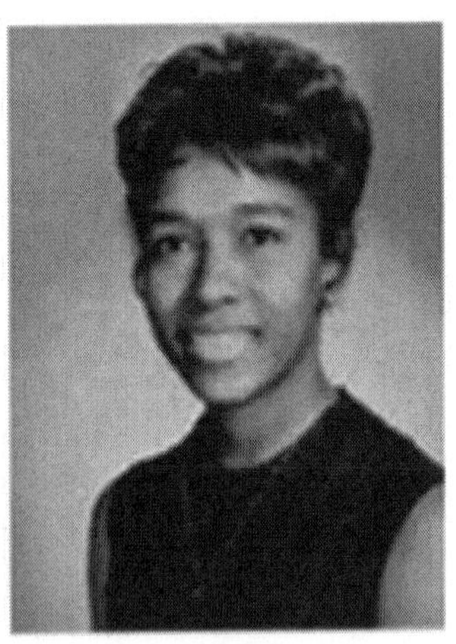

Norma Jenkins, B.S.
Howard University
1965

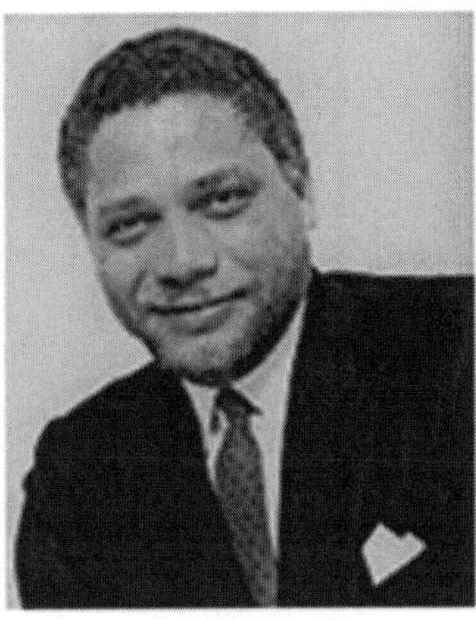

George T. Leland, B.S.
Texas Southern University
1970

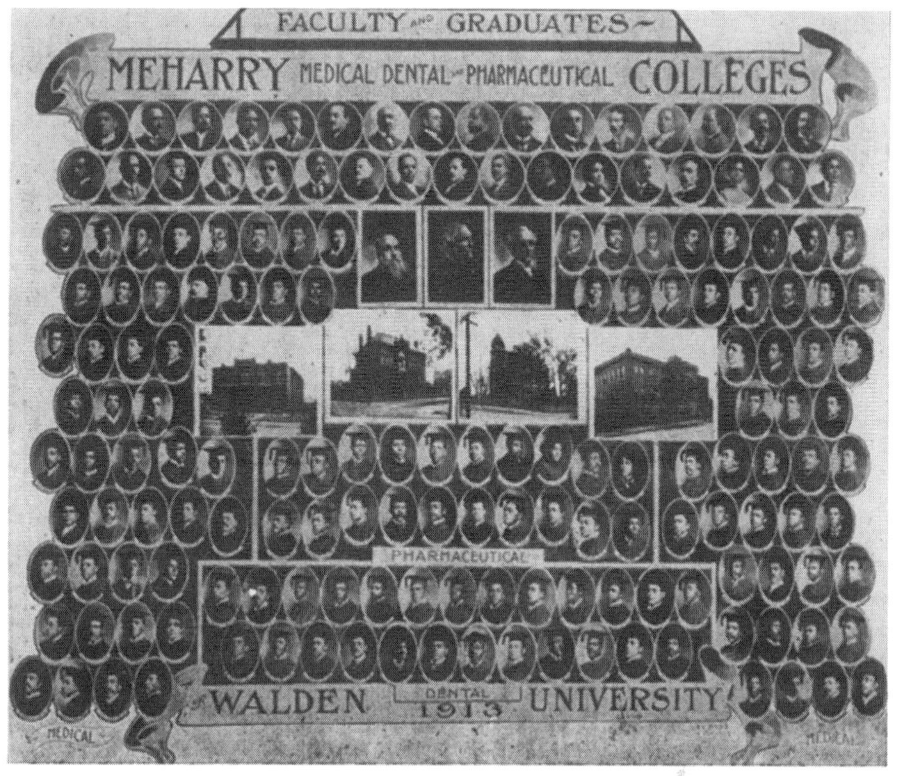

Meharry Medical College, Class of 1913.

(Source: *Nashville Globe*, April 25, 1913, p. 1.)

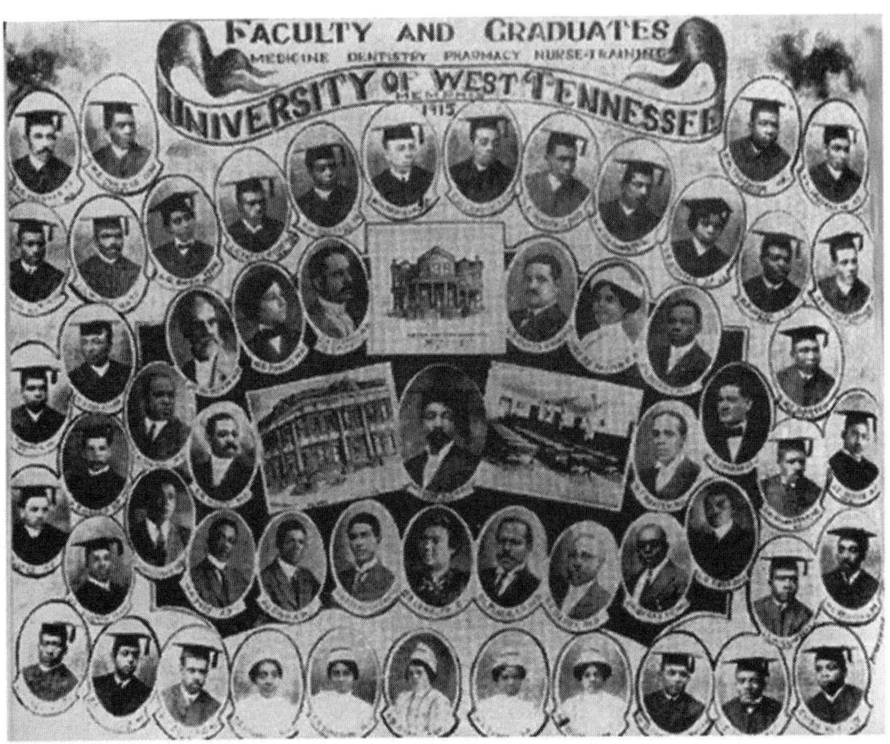

University of West Tennessee, Class of 1915.

(Source: Herbert M. Morais, *International Library of Negro Life and History: The History of the Negro in Medicine*, New York: Publishers Co., 1967.)

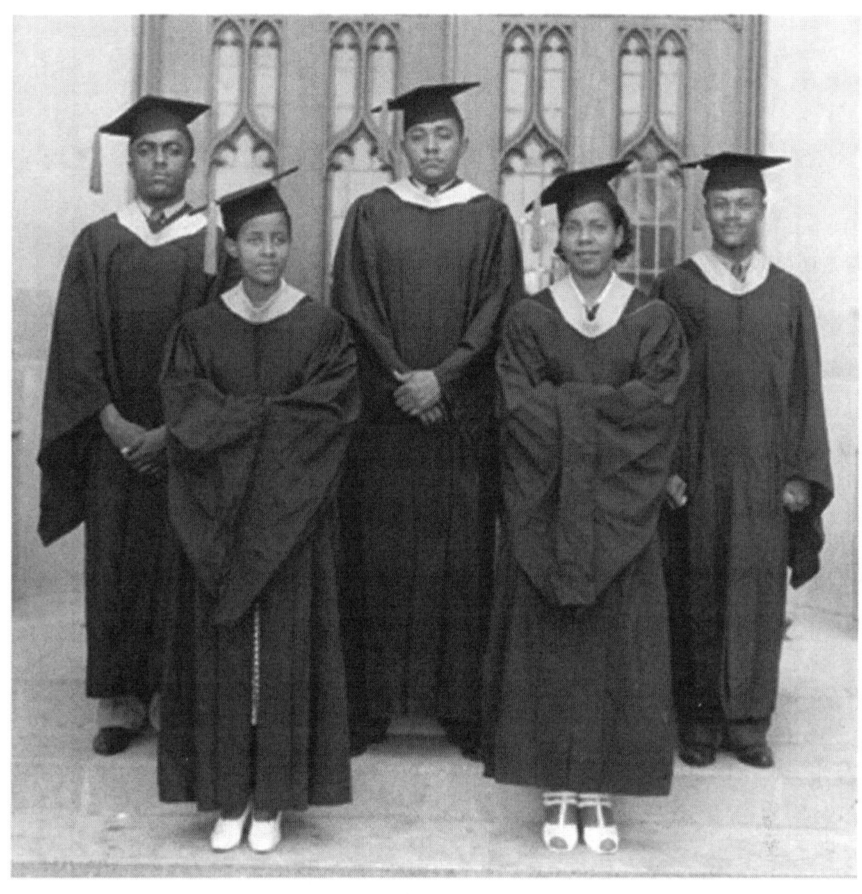

Xavier University College of Pharmacy Class of 1938. Front row: Pearl Inez Barnes (l), Thelma Rita Cunningham (r).

(Source: Xavier University of Louisiana, *Library Resources Center, Archives and Special Collections*.)

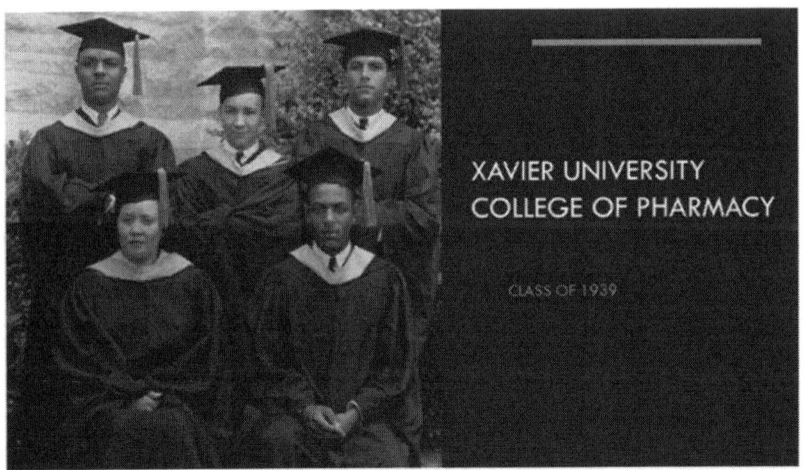

Xavier University College of Pharmacy Class of 1939.

(Source: Xavier University of Louisiana, *Library Resources Center, Archives and Special Collections*.)

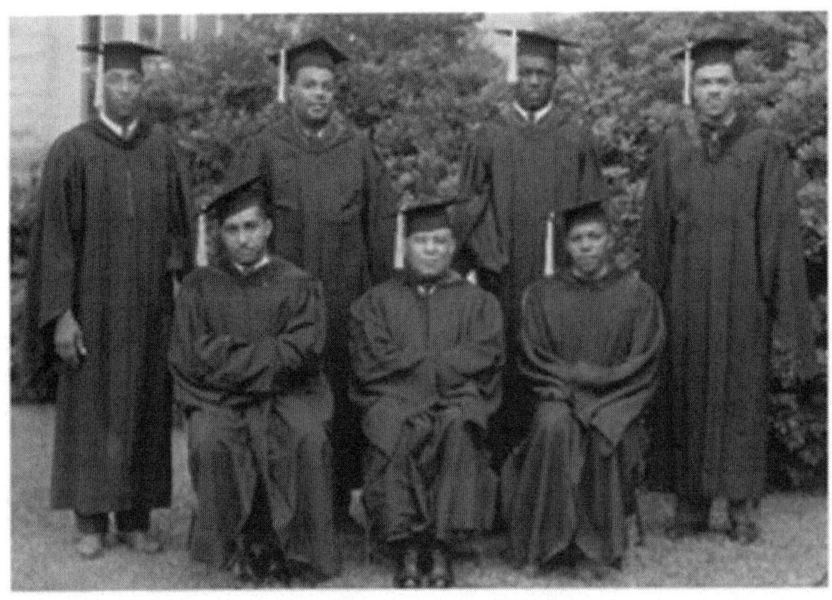

Xavier University College of Pharmacy Class of 1941.

(Source: Xavier University of Louisiana, *Library Resources Center, Archives and Special Collections*.)

Notes and References

1. U.S. Congress. House of Representatives. Office of the Historian. *History, Art & Archives, Women in Congress, 1917–2006.* Washington, D.C.: U.S. Government Printing Office, 2007; "The Women's Rights Movement, 1848–1920,", accessed October 05, 2015, http://history.house.gov/Exhibitions-and-Publications/WIC/Historical-Essays/No-Lady/Womens-Rights/; "Women's Suffrage in the United States." Wikipedia, The Free Encyclopedia. Wikimedia Foundation, Inc. Accessed October 18, 2015. https://en.wikipedia.org/wiki/Women%27s_suffrage_in_the_United_States

2. "The Negro in Pharmacy," *Drug Circular and Chemical Gazette* 41 (1897): 323.

3. Union Alumni Association, *Alumni Catalogue of Howard University with List of Incorporators, Trustees, and Other Employees. 1867-1896.* (Washington, DC: Howard University Print, 1896).

4. Washington College of Pharmacy was in existence from 1922-1926. It was a private, independent, proprietary school for African Americans, located in Washington, D.C. It is estimated to have graduated approximately 75 African American students before closing in 1926 amidst competition with other schools in the area and because of a lack of financial support. Catalogues and other information about the school was not located.

5. W. Michael Byrd and Linda A. Clayton. "An American Health Dilemma: A History of Blacks in the Health System," *Journal National Medical Association,* 84.2 (1992): 189-200. See also Margaret Humphreys, *Marrow of Tragedy: The Health Crisis of the American Civil War* (Baltimore, MD: Johns Hopkins University Press, 2013)

6. "Freedmen's Bureau Acts of 1865 and 1866." United States Senate. https://www.senate.gov/artandhistory/history/common/generic/FreedmensBureau.htm (accessed January 31, 2018); African American Heritage. "African American Records: Freedmen's Bureau." National Archives. https://www.archives.gov/research/african-americans/freedmens-bureau (accessed January 31, 2018).

7. Byrd and Clayton. "An American Health Dilemma" (n. 5). See also, W. Michael Byrd and Linda A. Clayton. *An American Health Dilemma: Race, Medicine, and Health Care in the United States, 1900-2000* (New York, NY: Routledge, 2002).

8. "Black Belt." *Encyclopedia Britannica. Encyclopedia Britannica Online.* Encyclopedia Britannica Inc., http://www.britannica.com/place/Black-Belt (accessed October 24, 2015).

9. U. S. Government Printing Office. (1993). *We the Americans: Blacks:* U.S. Department of Commerce Economics and Statistics Administration, Bureau of the Census. Washington, DC: Author.

10. Abraham Flexner, *Medical Education in the United States and Canada. A Report of the Carnegie Foundation for the Advancement of Teaching. Book Number Four*, (New York, NY: Carnegie Foundation for the Advancement of Teaching, 1910). http://archive.carnegiefoundation.org/pdfs/elibrary/Carnegie_Flexner_Report.pdf

11. Earl H. Harley, "The Forgotten History of Defunct Black Medical Schools in the 19th and 20th Centuries and the Impact of the Flexner Report." *Journal of the National Medical Association* 98.9 (September 2006): 1425-29; Robert B. Baker et. al., "Creating a Segregated Medical Profession: African American Physicians and Organized Medicine, 1846-1910." *Journal of the National Medical Association* 101.6 (June 2009): 501-12.

12. Wilbur H. Watson, *Against the Odds: Blacks in the Profession of Medicine in the United States* (New Brunswick, NJ: Transaction Publishers, 1999), 21.

13. Harriett A. Washington et.al. "Segregation, Civil Rights, and Health Disparities: The Legacy of African American Physicians and Organized Medicine, 1910-1968." *Journal of the National Medical Association.* 101.6 (June 2009): 513-527.

14. The medical colleges that were forced to close with pharmacy programs included: Shaw Leonard School of Medicine and Pharmacy, University of West Tennessee College of Physicians and Surgeons Department of Pharmacy, New Orleans University College of Pharmacy of Flint Medical College, and the Louisville National Medical College Department of Pharmacy.

15. Chauncey I. Cooper, "Section 12. The Negro in Pharmacy," in *The General Report of the Pharmaceutical Survey 1946-49,* ed. Edward C. Elliott (Washington, DC: American Council on Education, 1947), 181-187. See also, Dennis B. Worthen, "Chauncey Ira Cooper (1906–1983): Champion of Minority Pharmacists," *Journal American Pharmacists Association,* 46.1 (January/February): 100-103.

16. Chas H. Thompson, "Editorial Note. The Availability of Education in the Negro Separate School," *Journal of Negro Education* 16. No. 3 (Summer, 1947): 263-268.

17. *Civil Rights Act of 1964*. Public Law 88-352, Title VII, Sec. 703, 78. *U.S. Statutes at Large* (July 2, 1964).

18. *Morrill Act of 1862*, 7 U.S.C. § 301; *Higher Education Act of 1965*. Public Law 92-318, 79. *U.S. Statutes at Large* (November 8, 1965).

19. United States Department of Labor. Office of the Assistant Secretary for Administration and Management. *Title IX, Education Amendments of 1972,* accessed October 18, 2015, https://www.dol.gov/oasam/regs/statutes/titleix.htm; Richard Nixon: "Statement on Signing the Education Amendments of 1972.", June 23, 1972. Online by Gerhard Peters and John T. Woolley, *The American Presidency Project.* http://www.presidency.ucsb.edu/ws/?pid=3473.

20. *Higher Education Act of 1965* (n. 18); Federal Student Aid (FSA), Office of the U.S. Department of Education. https://studentaid.ed.gov/sa/about

21. Katherine K. Knapp and James M. Cultice, "New Pharmacist Supply Projections: Lower Separation Rates and Increased Graduates Boost Supply Estimates." *Journal American Pharmacists Association* 47.4 (2007): 463-470; *An Era of Growth and Change: A Closer Look at Pharmacy Education and Practice,* (Oakland, CA: The University of California Office of the President's Division of Health Sciences, February 2014), http://health.universityofcalifornia.edu/ ; Stephen F. Eckel, "The Value of a Pharmacy Education." *Pharmacy Times,* Retrieved March 12, 2014, http://www.pharmacytimes.com/publications/health-system-edition/2014/march2014/the-value-of-a-pharmacy-education; Ashish Advani, "Pharmacist Supply and Demand: Past, Present, and Future." *Pharmacy Times*, Retrieved October 28, 2014, http://www.pharmacytimes.com/contributor/dr-ashish-advani-pharmd/2014/10/pharmacist-supply-and-demand-past-present-and-future; Alex Barker, "The Pharmacy Job Crisis: Blame the Pharmacy School Bubble." *Pharmacy Times*, Retrieved May 26, 2015, http://www.pharmacytimes.com/contributor/alex-barker-pharmd/2015/05/the-pharmacy-job-crisis-blame-the-pharmacy-school-bubble.

22. Victor Yanchick, Jeffrey N. Baldwin, et. al., "AACP REPORTS: Report of the 2013-2014 Argus Commission: Diversity and Inclusion in Pharmacy Education," *American Journal of Pharmaceutical Education* 78 (2014): S21; Roland A. Patry, Lea S. Eland, "Addressing the Shortage of Pharmacy Faculty and Clinicians: The Impact of Demographic Changes." *American Journal Health-system Pharmacy* 64(April 1, 2007): 773-775; Hannah K. Vanderpool, "ASHP Report: Report of the ASHP Ad Hoc Committee on Ethnic Diversity and Cultural Competence." *American Journal Health-system Pharmacy* 62(September 15, 2005): 1924-1930; ASHP Report. "Report of the ASHP Task Force on Pharmacy's Changing Demographics." *American Journal Health-system Pharmacy* 64(June 15, 2007): 1311-1319.

23. Daniel Smith Lamb. *Howard University Medical Department, Washington, D.C.: A Historical, Biographical and Statistical Souvenir*. (Washington, DC: R. Beresford, 1900).

24. Walter Dyson. *Howard University the Capstone of Negro Education, A History: 1867-1940.* (Washington, D.C.: The Graduate School of Howard University, 1941).

25. Lamb, *Howard University Medical Department* (n. 23), 143.

26. Julia Pearl Hughes describes the opportunity that she was granted by the surgeon in chief at the Freedman's Hospital to gain experience in the hospital's drug store, where she worked daily during her two-year course of study in pharmacy school at Howard University from about 1895 until her graduation in 1897. See "The Negro in Pharmacy" (n. 2), p. 323. When she left the Frederick Douglas Memorial Hospital to open her own drugstore, she appeared in the pharmacy news, although some would think as being described in a derogatory manner, as being the first African American woman ("negress") to own a drugstore in the U.S. See also, "A Negress in Pharmacy," *Bulletin of Pharmacy*, 13.12 (1900): 484.

27. *Morrill Act of 1862*, 7 U.S.C. § 301 (1862); *Higher Education Act of 1965*. Public Law 92-318, 79. *U.S. Statutes at Large* (November 8, 1965).

28. "Separate but Equal Doctrine." West's Encyclopedia of American Law, edition 2. 2008. The Gale Group 19 Oct. 2015 http://legal-dictionary.thefreedictionary.com/Separate+but+Equal+Doctrine

29. Brad Lightcap, "The Morrill Act of 1862." http://www3.nd.edu/~rbarger/www7/morrill.html. Accessed December 23, 2016.

30. Land grant aid of colleges, 7 U.S.C. § 301 (1862); 26 Stat. 417; 7 U.S.C. § 321 (1890).

31. Land grant aid of colleges, (n. 30); "HBCUs and 2020 Goals," White House Initiative on Historically Black Colleges and Universities. U.S. Department of Education, http://sites.ed.gov/whhbcu/ Accessed October 24, 2015 (accessed October 24, 2015).

32. Freedmen's Aid Society. *Report of the Freedmen's Aid Society of the Methodist Episcopal Church.* (Cincinnati, OH: R.F. Thompson, Printers, 1868); Report on Freedmen's Aid. "Freedmen's Aid Society Methodist Episcopal Church History." Freedmen's Aid Society. http://www.drbronsontours.com/bronsonfreedmensaidsocietymethodistepiscopalchurchhistory.html (accessed January 31, 2018).

33. William C. Turner, "African-American Education in Eastern North Carolina: American Baptist Mission Work." *American Baptist Quarterly,* 12 (1992): 290-308. See also Clara Merritt DeBoer "Blacks and the American Missionary Association." *United Church of Christ.* http://www.ucc.org/about-us_hidden-histories_blacks-and-the-american (accessed January 31, 2018).

34. Chauncey I. Cooper, "Section 12. The Negro in Pharmacy," in *The General Report of the Pharmaceutical Survey 1946-49,* ed. Edward C. Elliott (Washington, DC: American Council on Education, 1947), 181-187.

35. *Civil Rights Act of 1866*, 18 Stat. 27-30 (1866).

36. *Civil Rights Act of 1875*, 18 Stat. 335-337 (1875); also known as the Enforcement Act or Force Act.

37. *Civil Rights Act of 1875*, (n. 36); Wormser, Richard. "Civil Rights Act of 1875 Declared Unconstitutional." Jim Crow Stories. Accessed March 18, 2018. https://www.thirteen.org/wnet/jimcrow/stories_events_uncivil.html

38. "Homer Adolph Plessy ", A Dictionary of Louisiana Biography, Vol. 2 (1988), p.655, http://en.academic.ru/dic.nsf/enwiki/553859 (accessed October 24, 2015); *Plessy vs Ferguson*, 163 US 537 (1896), https://supreme.justia.com/cases/federal/us/163/537/case.html (accessed October 24, 2015).

39. "Separate but Equal Doctrine." (n. 28); Harry E. Groves, "Separate but Equal–The Doctrine of Plessy v. Ferguson". *Phylon* 12.1 (1915): 66–72.

40. "Louisiana 'Jim Crow' Law Valid." *New York Times* 21 December 1892; Klarman, Michael J. *From Jim Crow to Civil Rights: The Supreme Court and the Struggle for Racial Equality*. (New York, NY: Oxford University Press, 2004).

41. "The Shame of America." *New York Times,* November 23, 1922. http://www.digitalhistory.uh.edu/active_learning/explorations/lynching/shame.cfm. See also, Work, M. Nathan. *Negro Year Book: An Annual Encyclopedia of the Negro ...1947,1952.* (Tuskegee Institute, Ala.: Negro Year Book Pub. Co., 1912).

42. "Wins Discrimination Suit Against Railway," *The New York Age,* \July 6, 1918. Many African Americans, regardless of education, could not vote in some states until after 1960, but also could not simply sit where they please while taking public transportation. See Ann D. Gordon and Bettye Collier-Thomas, Bettye. *African American Women and the Vote, 1837-1965* (Amherst, MA: University of Massachusetts Press, 1997). Because of the *Plessy vs Ferguson* decision, railways often created separate riding coaches and the law made it illegal for black passengers to sit in coaches designated for white passengers. In cases where lawsuits were filed, and won by black passengers, the awards were very nominal, at times as low as one cent. The legal action rarely changed the law or the practice. See also "Verdict for One Cent – Colored Lawyer, in 'Jim Crow' Suit Awarded Nominal Damages." *The Washington Post,* May 16, 1907, 13.

43. "Negro Passenger Sues Rock Island," *The Des Moines Register*, April 15, 1950, 3.

44. Addie W. Hunton and Kathryn M. Johnson, *Two Colored Women with the American Expeditionary Forces* (Brooklyn, NY: Brooklyn Eagle Press, 1920), 57-61. Matthew Virgil Boutte was a 1911 graduate of the University of Illinois College of Pharmacy (Ph.C., Ph.G.) and former faculty member of the Meharry Medical College. He was fluent in the French and English languages. He

would serve as interpreter for the soldiers during World War I while in France; See "John D. Rockefeller Jr. Delivers His First Commencement Address at 1928 Commencement, Fisk University," *New York Age,* June 16, 1928, 2. Because he became friends with some of French citizens, his supervising officer ordered him "not to take the French people's kindness for friendship, but to treat them just as he had been taught to treat white people at home. When they found that his ability to speak French gave him ready entrée into French homes, they relieved him of all work as billeting officer, so that he would have no occasion for going among the French people. While under arrest he was forced to ride from one town to another in an open wagon, and between two armed guards, and with no weapon to protect himself if they came under fire, in order that his spirit might be thoroughly crushed and humiliated."

45. Prior to World War I, Matthew Boutte had the experience of operating the Northside Pharmacy in Nashville, Tennessee. After the war ended, he and his wife, pharmacist Etnah R. Boutte, opened Boutte's Pharmacy in New York, which was reported to have over $10,000 in pharmaceutical inventory and generated over $50,000 a year in gross revenue. See "Boutte's Pharmacy." *The Crisis*. November 1925, 24; See also "Mathieu V. Boutte Buried at Arlington," *New York Age,* October 19, 1957, p. 3.

46. "28 Netters Expected in Chickasaw Meet." *Courier-Journal,* May 29, 1958; "Idle Hour Club Bars Negro Tennis Player." *Advocate-Messenger*, August 1, 1958; "Paniello and Daus Gain in State Play." *Courier-Journal*, July 31, 1958; "Baughman Brothers Advance in State Tourney, Lexington." *Interior Journal*, August 1, 1958.

47. Zirl A. Palmer, his wife, and 4-year old daughter were severely injured from the bomb blast. Phillip J. Campbell, a former member of the Ku Klux Klan, was sentenced to 21 years in prison for the attack. The motive for the attack was because of Palmer's business success and his involvement in civil rights activities, which included organizing voter's registration drives, an anti-poverty agency, and leading the Lexington Human Rights Commission. See Phil Norman. "Bomb Victim Suspects Anti-Rights Terrorism." *Courier-Journal*, September 6, 1968; "3 Business Demolished by Explosion." *Messenger-Inquirer*, September 5, 1968; "Blast Rocks Supermarket at Lexington." *Cincinnati Enquirer*, September 5, 1968.

48. "Mr. Nixon and the Revolution." *Courier-Journal,* August 30, 1972; "First Black UK Trustee, Zirl Palmer, Dies at 62." *Courier-Journal,* May 21, 1982. For more incidents involving Zirl Palmer, see his interview at: https://kentuckyoralhistory.org/ark:/16417/xt7vt43j136n

49. "What the Negro is Doing: Matters of Interest Among the Colored People." *The Atlanta Constitution*. October 31, 1897, 32; "They Say That," *Drug Circular and Chemical Gazette* 41 (March 1897): 28.

50. John J. Mullowney, "What Future is There for the Negro Pharmacist?" *Journal of National Medical Association* 24, no. 3 (1932): 27-29.

51. F. Marion Fletcher, *The Racial Policies of American Industry, Report No. 24, The Negro the Drugstore Industry,* (Philadelphia, PA: University of Pennsylvania Press, 1970), 24.

52. Robert W. Culp, *The Genesis of Black Pharmacists in America to 1900* (Unknown Binding, 1975); "The Negro in Pharmacy" (n. 2), p. 323; "The Women's Rights Movement" (n. 1); Editorial. *The Druggist* 6.1 (January 1884): 15; "National College of Pharmacy." *American Druggist,* 13 (1884): 11; "Color Line in Alabama." *Pharmaceutical Era.* 13 (May 30, 1895): 674; "The Color Line in Pharmacy." *Pharmaceutical Era.* 15 (1896): 637-638.

53. "Notes and Queries," *Drug Circular and Chemical Gazette* 171 (1873): 111. "The Color Line in Pharmacy" (n. 52), p. 637-638.

54. "The Negro in Pharmacy" (n. 2), p. 323.

55. "The Negro in Pharmacy" (n. 2), p. 323.

56. "African Americans in the Pharmaceutical Profession in the Mid-20th Century," in *United States Department of the Interior. National Park Service / National Register of Historic Places Registration Form.* NPS Form 10-900. OMB No. 1024-0018. Green Valley Pharmacy. Arlington, VA.

57. "African Americans in the Pharmaceutical Profession in the Mid-20th Century," (n. 56); "The Color Line in Pharmacy" (n. 52). For decades, white drug store owners would not service African-American patrons at their soda fountains and thus their drug stores became one of the major targets where protest took place throughout the 1960s' Civil Rights movement. See Booker, Jamal. "Fighting for Civil Rights at the Soda Fountain." http://www.coca-colacompany.com/history/fighting-for-civil-rights-at-the-soda-fountain (accessed January 14, 2018).

58. "Colored People Apparently Prefer to Patronize White Druggists." *The Indianapolis News*, January 18, 1904, 11; Carter Godwin Woodson, "Pharmacists as They Function," in *The Negro Professional Man and the Community,* ed. Carter G. Woodson (Washington, D.C.: The Association for the Study of Negro Life and History, Inc., 1934), 149-164.

59. Culp, *The Genesis of Black Pharmacists* (n. 52); Nicole Carmolingo, "Henry Rutherford Butler (1862-1931)" New *Georgia Encyclopedia,* accessed April 24, 2016, http://www.georgiaencyclopedia.org/articles/science-medicine/henry-rutherford-butler-1862-1931.

60. Culp, *The Genesis of Black Pharmacists* (n. 52); "The Negro in Pharmacy" (n. 2); "The Color line in Pharmacy," (n. 52).

61. Mullowney, "What Future is There for the Negro Pharmacist?" (n. 51), p. 27; "The Negro in Pharmacy" (n. 2), p. 323.

62. Fletcher, *The Negro the Drugstore Industry* (n. 49).

63. Mullowney, "What Future is There for the Negro Pharmacist?" (n. 51), p. 27.

64. Phillip A. White received a diploma in pharmacy from the City College of New York in 1844. He later opened a drug store in New York in partnership with Dr. James McCune Smith, a physician and pharmacist, whom he had completed his pharmacy apprenticeship. See the College of Pharmacy of the City of New York, *Prospectus of the College of Pharmacy of the City of New York, Forty-First Session, October 1870 to March 1871*, (New York: Brown & Co., Stationers and Printers, 1870); Culp. *The Genesis of Black Pharmacists in America to 1900*, (n. 52).

65. "The Negro in Pharmacy" (n. 2), p. 323.

66. *Columbia University, Bulletin of Information, College of Pharmacy of the City of New York*, (New York, NY: Columbia University, 1921).

67. *Columbia University Bulletin of Information, College of Pharmacy of the City of New York included in Columbia University July 1, 1904, 1914-1915,* (New York: Columbia University, 1915).

68. *Columbia University Bulletin of Information. College of Pharmacy of the City of New York, Announcement 1924-1925, Twenty-fourth Series, No. 49* (New York, NY: Columbia University, 1924), 61; "Three Negroes Among Graduates of Columbia College of Pharmacy," *New York Age*, May 26, 1923, 1.

69. *The Apothekan, College of Pharmacy of the City of New York, Class of 1927,* (New York: F. J. Pokorny, 1927).

70. Frank L. Mather, *Who's Who of the Colored Race: A General Biographical Dictionary of Men and Women of African Descent, Volume One 1915*, (Chicago, IL: Frank Lincoln Mather, 1915), 24.

71. *Fiftieth Annual Announcement, University of Illinois School of Pharmacy, Chicago College of Pharmacy, Session of 1909 and 1910,* (Chicago: University of Illinois, 1910); Mather, *Who's Who of the Colored Race* (n. 71), p. 31; "School of Pharmacy (U. Ill.) Notes," *NARD Journal* 28.6 (May 1919): 286

72. University of Illinois, *The Illio Yearbook,* 1912, 466.

73. *School of Pharmacy of the University of Michigan, Register of Alumni and Announcement, Twenty-six Year, 1893-1894,* (Ann Arbor: University of Michigan, 1893); *Memphis Biography*: George R. Jackson. Nashville, TN: Tennessee Historical Commission, 1990.

74. *School of Pharmacy of the University of Michigan, Register of Alumni and Announcement, Twenty-six Year, 1901-1902,* (Ann Arbor: University of Michigan, 1901).

75. *University of Michigan School of Pharmacy Announcement for 1909-1910,* (Ann Arbor: University of Michigan, 1910).

76. *University of Michigan School of Pharmacy Announcement for 1922-1923,* (Ann Arbor: University of Michigan, 1923).

77. "Classes of the Philadelphia College of Pharmacy, Seventy-Fourth Annual Session, 1894-1895," *American Journal of Pharmacy* 67 (January 1895): 285; M. Van Houten. "Minto, Henry McKee (1870-1946)," *BlackPast.org*, accessed April 24, 2016, http://www.blackpast.org/aah/minton-henry-mckee-1870-1946.

78. Joseph W. England, *The First Century of the Philadelphia College of Pharmacy, 1821-1921* (Philadelphia, PA: Philadelphia College of Pharmacy, 1922), 641, 684; Thomas Yenser, *Who's Who in Colored America. A Biographical Dictionary of Notable Living Persons of African Descent in America. 1941-19445, 6th ed.* (Brooklyn, NY: Who's Who in Colored America, 1940).

79. "The Negro in Pharmacy," (n. 2), p. 323; "New Jersey Negro Pharmacist." *The Druggists Circular and Chemical Gazette* 41 (December 1897): 369.

80. Dubois, W.E.B. "Colleges and Their Graduates." In *The Crisis. A record of the Darker Races, November 1923 – October 1924.* Authorized reprint ed. New York: ARNO Press, 1969, p. 113, 114.

81. *The Brooklyn College of Pharmacy Sixth Annual Announcement, Session of 1896-97*, (Brooklyn, NY: Brooklyn College of Pharmacy, 1897), p. 29.

82. *The Brooklyn College of Pharmacy Sixth Annual Announcement*, (n. 64), p. 29.

83. *Brooklyn College of Pharmacy, The Brooklyn College of Pharmacy Twentieth Annual Announcement, Session of 1910-1911.* (Brooklyn, New York: Eagle Press, 1911).

84. Gregory Bond, "Recovering and Expanding Mozella Esther Lewis's Pioneering History of African-American Pharmacy Students, 1870-1925," *Pharmacy in History* 58.1.2 (2016): 3-23.

85. "Mrs. Hattie Hutchinson," *The Bystander,* September 11, 1908, 1.

86. *Temple University, The Temple University Bulletin, Annual Catalogue 1911-1912.* (Philadelphia, PA: Temple University, 1911). Accessed January 15, 2016. http://hdl.handle.net/2027/uiug.30112111450356 15 January 2016. Three African American females started in the same class, which may have been a first, but only two are listed in the graduating class of 1911. The third was Chesta Dillard Dean.

87. *The Yearbook of the Department of Pharmacy, Class of 1916, Temple University.* (Philadelphia, PA: Temple University, 1916).

88. *The Temple University Bulletin, Annual Catalogue, Volume 1, May 1919,* (Philadelphia, PA: Temple University, 1919).

89. "Negro in Higher Education 1921-22," *The Crisis, A Record of the Darker Races* 23.1 (November 1921): 112

90. W.E.B. Dubois, "Colored Students and Graduates 1923," *The Crisis* 26.3 (July 1923): 110.

91. *The Pharmacopian, Class of 1926, Temple University Sesqui Centennial Pharmacy Class,* (Philadelphia, PA: Majestic Press, 1926).

92. *University of Washington, Catalogue of the University of Washington for 1912-1913 and Announcements for 1913-1914* (Olympia, WA: Frank M. Lamborn Public Printer, 1913), p. 332; *University of Washington, Catalogue of the University of Washington for 1914-1915 and Announcements for 1915-1916* (Olympia, WA: Frank M. Lamborn Public Printer, 1915). Alice Augusta Ball went on to discover a treatment for leprosy. See also "Alice Ball: The Unsung Black Chemist Who Fought Leprosy," Rejected Princesses.com. http://www.rejectedprincesses.com/blog/modern-worthies/alice-ball (accessed January 16, 2018).

93. *University of Washington, Catalogue of the University of Washington for 1915-1916 and Announcements for 1916-1917* (Olympia, WA: Frank M. Lamborn Public Printer, 1917); *University of Washington, Catalogue of the University of Washington for 1921-1922 and Announcements for 1922-1923* (Seattle: University of Washington Press, 1922).

94. *The University of Minnesota Bulletin, College of Pharmacy 1909-1910, Volume XII, No. 3, April 1909* (Minneapolis, MN: University of Minnesota, 1909), pp. 3, 35; *The University of Minnesota, The College of Pharmacy 1912-1913. Bulletin of the University of Minnesota, Volume XV, No. 3, May 1912* (Minneapolis, MN: University of Minnesota, 1912).

95. *Bulletin of the University of Minnesota*, 1912 (n. 77), p.34.

96. *The University of Minnesota, The College of Pharmacy 1915-1916. Bulletin of the University of Minnesota, Volume XVIII, No. 10, May 1915* (Minneapolis, MN: University of Minnesota, 1915), p. 22.

97. *Bulletin of the University of Minnesota, The Annual Register, Vol. XLX No. 2, April 1918,* (Minneapolis, MN: University of Minnesota, 1918), 123.

98. *University of Pittsburgh, Annual Catalog, 1913-1914, University of Pittsburgh Year Ending June 1914* (Pittsburgh, PA: Murdoch, Kerr & Co., 1914); W. E. B. Dubois, "Colleges and Their Graduates in 1914," *The Crisis* 8.1 (May 1914): 133-140

99. *University of Pittsburgh, Annual Catalog, 1915-1916, University of Pittsburgh Year Ending June 1916.* (Pittsburgh, PA: Murdoch, Kerr & Co, 1916); *Annual Catalog University of Pittsburgh Ninety-Seventh Year, 1916-1917* (Pittsburgh, PA: Smith Bros. Company Inc., 1917).

100. Gregory Bond. "Yet in All This Library There is Scarcely a Reference to the Negro in Pharmacy:" The University of Wisconsin's Leo Butts, Pioneering Historian of African-American Pharmacists" *Pharmacy in History* 59.1&2

(2017): 34-46; *Bulletin of the University of Wisconsin, The University of Wisconsin Catalogue 1919-20* (Madison: University of Wisconsin, 1920), p. 538.

101. *The State University of Iowa Calendar 1906-1907* (Iowa City: University of Iowa, 1907), p. 565; *The State University of Iowa Calendar 1907-1908, Including the Announcements for 1908-1909* (Iowa City: University of Iowa, 1908), p. 532.

102. *The State University of Iowa Calendar 1909-1910, Including the Announcements for 1910-1911* (Iowa City: University of Iowa, 1910), p. 402. George O. Caldwell received the National Dispensatory Prize award in 1909 as a member of the senior class who presented the best paper before the Iowa Alumni Association. See also *The State University of Iowa, Announcement of the College of Pharmacy 1910-1911* (Iowa City: University of Iowa, 1910), p. 13.

103. *The State University of Iowa. Catalogue 1921-1922 - including Announcements for 1922-1923* (Iowa City, IA: University of Iowa, 1923), 500.

104. *The Makio,* (Columbus, OH: Ohio State University, 1897) 112-113.

105. *The Makio,* (Columbus, OH: Ohio State University, 1913) 207.

106. *The Ohio State University Catalogue 1921-1922, Announcement 1922-1923* (Columbus: Ohio State University, 1921), p. 436; "Negro in Higher Education 1921-22," (n. 61), p. 112.

107. Bond, "Recovering and Expanding Mozella Lewis" (n. 84) p. 13.

108. Bond, "Recovering and Expanding Mozella Lewis" (n. 84).

109. "Diplomas to 38 – Massachusetts College of Pharmacy Graduates – One Young Women receives Degree," *The Boston Daily Globe*, May 21, 1915, 15; "M.C.P. Commencement," *The Spatula*, 21.9 (June 1915): 474; "Colleges Graduate Many New Pharmacists – Massachusetts," *The Pharmaceutical Era,* 48.7 (July 1915): 324.

110. Bond, "Recovering and Expanding Mozella Lewis" (n. 84) p. 843; "Negro in Higher Education 1921-22," (n. 61), p. 112, 113.

111. "Mary Brickson Hill: A Pioneer at MCPHS, *MCHPS University Alumni & Friends,* October 9, 2019, https://www.alumni.mcphs.edu/s/1022/18/interior.aspx?sid=1022&gid=1&pgid=252&cid=6160&ecid=6160&crid=0&calpgid=1547&calcid=3720

112. *Western Reserve University in the City of Cleveland Catalogue 1920-1921* (Cleveland: Western Reserve University, 1922), p. 417; Bond, "Recovering and Expanding Mozella Lewis" (n. 84) p. 17.

113. Bond, "Recovering and Expanding Mozella Lewis" (n. 84) p. 17; *Third Annual Announcement of the Buffalo College of Pharmacy, Department of Pharmacy*

University of Buffalo, Session of 1915-1916 (Buffalo: University of Buffalo, 1916), p. 42.

114. *The Griffin, 1927 Yearbook of the College of the City of Detroit* (Detroit, MI: College of the City of Detroit, 1927), 15.

115. *The Griffin, 1928 Yearbook of the College of the City of Detroit* (Detroit, MI: College of the City of Detroit, 1928), 78.

116. *The Griffin, 1930 Yearbook of the College of the City of Detroit* (Detroit, MI: College of the City of Detroit, 1930), 40.

117. *The Griffin, 1932 Yearbook of the College of the City of Detroit* (Detroit, MI: College of the City of Detroit, 1932), 123.

118. Editorial. *The Druggist* 6.1 (January 1884): 15; "National College of Pharmacy." *American Druggist,* 13 (1884): 11.

119. Editorial (n. 118), p. 15.

120. *Alumni Catalogue of Howard University* (n. 3), 24; Roy C. Darlington, *A History of Pharmaceutical Education at Howard University 1868-1981* (Washington DC: Howard University, 2016). Dr. Oliver Atwood also received a medical degree (M.D.) at Howard and went on to practice medicine in Washington, D.C. for many years. See also Ancestry.com. *U.S. City Directories, 1822-1995* [database on-line]. Provo, UT, USA: Ancestry.com Operations, Inc. 2011.

121. "Mrs. Hattie Hutchinson," *The Bystander,* December 6, 1907, 5; "248 To Finish at Highland Park," *The Des Moines Register,* July 19, 1908, 4.

122. "Pres. Bell Denies Drawing Color Line," *The Des Moines Register,* September 11, 1908, 10; "An Iowa College Draws Color Line," *Jackson Daily News,* September 12, 1908, 1; "Draws Color Line," *The Topeka State Journal,* September 12, 1908, 11; "Draws Color Line in Iowa College," *Oakland Tribune,* September 13, 1908, 26; "The Color Line Drawn at Highland Park, in Des Moines, IA," *New-State Tribune,* September 24, 1908, 4.

123. News. *The Bystander,* September 11, 1908, 1.

124. "Des Moines University College of Pharmacy," *Northwestern Druggist* 29 (July 1921): 78.

125. Jacqueline Jones Royester, "Ella Nora Phillips Myers Stewart." In *Profiles of Ohio Women, 1803 –2003,* (Athens, Ohio: Ohio University, 2003), 97; "Ella Stewart." *Contemporary Black Biography*. Vol. 39. Detroit: Gale, 2003. Accessed via Gale Biography in Context October 20, 2015. http://www.encyclopedia.com/education/news-wires-white-papers-and-books/stewart-ella-1893-1987; "Ella P. Stewart." Blue Gold & Black, University of Pittsburgh, Chancellor Mark A. Nordenberg Reports on the Pitt

African American Experience, 2010. Retrieved October 15, 2016. http://www.chancellor-emeritus.pitt.edu/sites/default/files/pdfs/2010-BGB.pdf

126. "Ella P. Stewart." Blue Gold & Black (n. 125).

127. *University of Pittsburgh, Annual Catalog, 1913-1914,* (n. 98).

128. *University of Pittsburgh, Annual Catalog, 1915-1916,* (n. 99).

129. Eugene Fauntleroy Cordell, *University of Maryland 1807-1907, Its History, Influence, Equipment and Characteristics with Biographical Sketches and Portraits of its Founders, Benefactors, Regents, Faculty and Alumni,* (New York: The Lewis Publishing Company, 1907), 405-454.

130. "Negro Student Sues to Enter U. of M. School," *The Baltimore Sun*, September 18, 1948, 24; "Court Asked to Help Negro Enter School," *Wilkes-Barre Times Leader,* September 20, 1948, 4; "Negro Groups to be Heard on Admission to U. of M.," *The Baltimore Sun,* September 2, 1948, 7.

131. "U. of M. Denies Race is a Basis for Rejection," *The Baltimore Sun,* October 23, 1948, 24

132. U. of M. Denies Race is a Basis for Rejection," (n. 131).

133. "Morgan Lists 231 Graduates," *The Baltimore Sun,* June 4, 1950, 24.

134. *Howard University Bulletin, The College of Medicine 1955-1956, With Announcements for 1956-1957 Sessions,* Washington DC: Howard University, 1955), 56. See also, "Physicians are Licensed," *The Baltimore Sun,* July 28, 1955, 11.

135. "Notable Deaths in the Washington Area," *The Washington Post,* May 9, 2014.

136. "Files Suit Against University of Maryland," *The News (Frederick Maryland),* July 26, 1949, 7; "6 Suits Filed to Gain Graduate Admission to Maryland University," *Alabama Tribune,* August 5, 1949, 5; "Suits to Force School to Accept Negroes Filed." *Leader-Telegram,* July 29, 1949, 24.

137. "2 More Negroes Charge U. of M." *The Baltimore Sun*, July 27, 1949, 28; "Answer to Negro Suits Ordered," *The Evening Sun*, August 1, 1949, 11.

138. James E. Hodges was the first African American graduate of the University of Maryland College of Pharmacy. He received the B.S. degree in 1957. See the *Terra Mariae,* University of Maryland Yearbook, 1957.

139. Cooper, "The Negro in Pharmacy" (n. 34).

140. "Separate but Equal Doctrine." (n. 39).

141. Chas. H. Thompson, "Editorial Note: The Availability of Education in the Negro Separate School," *The Journal of Negro Education,* 16.3 (Summer 1947): 263-268.

142. Hocutt v. Wilson, *N.C. Super. Ct.* (1933); See also, Jerry Gershenhorn, "Hocutt v. Wilson and Race Relations in Durham, North Carolina, During the 1930s," *The North Carolina Office of Archives and History,* 78.3 (July 2001): 275-308.

143. "Jim Crow School Test is Up Friday," *The Pittsburgh Courier,* March 25, 1933,1.

144. "Applicant for Admission to School of Pharmacy Files Writ of Mandamus – Lawyers Threaten to Take Case to Higher Courts if Necessary," *The Pittsburgh Courier,* March 25, 1933, 2; "Court Says School Must Show Cause of Ban of Negro," *The Pittsburgh Courier,* April 1, 1933, 13.

145. "Technicality is 'Hitch' as First Legal Clash Fails," *The Pittsburgh Courier,* April 8, 1933, 2; "Negro Youth Loses First Round of His Legal Battle Against University of North Carolina." *The New York Age,* April 8, 1933, 1.

146. "Negro's Suit to Get Into U-T up March 22," *The Knoxville News-Sentinel,* February 28, 1937, 17; "Racial School Ban Contested," *The Knoxville Journal,* February 28, 1937, 3; "Negro Demands Entry to Pharmacy School," *The Bristol Herald Courier,* February 28, 1937, 5; "Negro Student Seeks Entrance to State Varsity," *The Jackson Sun,* March 23, 1937, 2; "Negro is Suing to Enter U-T," *The Knoxville Journal,* March 22, 1937, 3.

147. "Negro Asks Right to Enter College Class for Whites," *Johnson City Press and Staff-News,* February 28, 1937, 20; "U-T Color Line Case Up Today," *The Knoxville News-Sentinel*, March 22, 1937, *3;* "Demand of Negro for Admission to U.T. Under Study," *Johnson City Press and Staff-News,* March 22, 1937, 1.

148. "Negro Denied U-T Entrance," The Knoxville Journal, April 17, 1937, 1; "Nashville Negro Denied Entrance to U-T School," *Johnson City Chronicle,* April 17, 1937, 1; "Bejach's Opinion, *The Knoxville Journal,* April 18, 1933, 4; "School's Refusal of Negro Upheld," *The Birmingham News,* April 17, 1937, 9.

149. "Dry Leadership in State Gird for Election Fight," *The Jackson Sun,* May 23, 1937, 2; "Examinations Are to Be Given for Negro Students." *The Jackson Sun*, September 16, 1937, 12; "Scholarship Exams for Negroes Slated," *Johnson City Press and State-News,* September 16, 13; "Negro School Aid Given by Scholarships," *The Knoxville Journal,* September 14, 1937, 11.

150. "First to Fight for Integration," *The Pittsburgh Courier,* June 26, 1954, 20; "Hocutt v. Wilson and Race Relations in Durham" (n. 142).

151. "Hocutt v. Wilson and Race Relations in Durham" (n. 142).

152. "Hocutt v. Wilson and Race Relations in Durham" (n. 142); "Kentucky Bars Negro," *The Pittsburgh Courier,* April 3, 1948, 5.

153. "Educational Equality Fight Shows Gains," *The Pittsburgh Courier,* October 21, 1950, 2.

154. "New NAACP Battle Against U. of Tenn.," *The Pittsburgh Courier,* March 24, 1951, 18; "Supreme Court's Decision Spurs Education Drive," *The Pittsburgh Courier,* December 24, 1938, 11; "Tenn. U. Campus Looks Over Gray," *The Pittsburgh Courier,* January 26, 1952, 19; "Equal Opportunity," *The Daily Tar Heel,* January 8, 1939.

155. *Yackety Yack Yearbook,* (Chapel Hill, NC: University of North Carolina, 1962).

156. *Yackety Yack Yearbook,* (Chapel Hill, NC: University of North Carolina, 1967).

157. *Ole Miss Yearbook* (Oxford, MS: University of Mississippi, 1970).

158. *Ole Miss Yearbook* (Oxford, MS: University of Mississippi, 1970).

159. *Ole Miss Yearbook* (Oxford, MS: University of Mississippi, 1975).

160. *Ole Miss Yearbook* (Oxford, MS: University of Mississippi, 1976).

161. *Ole Miss Yearbook* (Oxford, MS: University of Mississippi, 1973).

162. *Ole Miss Yearbook* (Oxford, MS: University of Mississippi, 1974).

163. *Ole Miss Yearbook* (Oxford, MS: University of Mississippi, 1975).

164. Helen Adams, "Pharmacist Dispenses Personal History Lesson for Black History Month," *MUSC News,* February 24, 2017, https://education.musc.edu/news/2017/02/24/black-history-month-pharmacist

165. *Entre Nous* (Birmingham, AL: Samford University, 1971).

166. *Entre Nous* (Birmingham, AL: Samford University, 1972).

167. *Entre Nous* (Birmingham, AL: Samford University, 1973)

168. Kasey Watkins, "Black History Month Feature: Phyllis Washington Gosa," *HSOP News*, February 26, 2015, http://www.auburn.edu/academic/pharmacy/news_events/2014-15/022615-gosa.html

169. "Linwood Moore: Part of Auburn's History," *HSOP News,* September 7, 2018, http://www.auburn.edu/academic/pharmacy/news_events/2018-19/0900718-linwood-moore.html

170. *Pandora Yearbook* (Athens, GA: University of Georgia, 1969), 360.

171. *Pandora Yearbook* (Athens, GA: University of Georgia, 1971), 364, 365.

172. *Pandora Yearbook* (Athens, GA: University of Georgia, 1972), 350.

173. *Pandora Yearbook* (Athens, GA: University of Georgia, 1973), 221.

174. "African American Undergraduates at the University of Kentucky," *Notable Kentucky African American Database NKAA,* October 12, 2019, https://nkaa.uky.edu/nkaa/items/show/3107

175. "History of the College of Pharmacy," *University of Tennessee Health Science Center,* October 17, 2019, https://www.uthsc.edu/pharmacy/about/history.php

176. *Caduceus Yearbook*, (Little Rock, AR: University of Arkansas for Medical Sciences, 1957), 101.

177. *Caduceus Yearbook*, (Little Rock, AR: University of Arkansas for Medical Sciences, 1961), 137.

178. Cooper, "The Negro in Pharmacy" (n. 34).

179. Roy C. Darlington. *A History of Pharmaceutical Education at Howard University, 1868-1981* (Washington, DC: Howard University College of Pharmacy, 2016); See also Xavier College Bulletins, 1929-1940. *Xavier University Bulletin, General Catalogue Number for the Academic Years: 1941-1950.* (New Orleans, L.A.: Sisters of the Blessed Sacrament, 1950).

180. "Walden University," *The Nashville Globe,* December 13, 1912, 10; "Facts and Figures That Tell the Story of Meharry Medical College, Nashville, Tenn." *The Nashville Globe,* April 25, 1913, 2.

181. "Walden University" (n. 180).

182. "Walden University" (n. 180); "Facts and Figures That Tell the Story of Meharry Medical College" (n. 180). For a more detailed history of the Meharry family, see Jessie Crawford Butler, et.al. *History of the Meharry Family in America: Descendants of Alexander Meharry I, Who Fled During the Reign of Mary Stuart, Queen of Scots, on Account of Religious Persecution, From Near Ayr, Scotland, to Ballyjamesduff, Cavan County, Ireland; and Whose Descendant Alexander Meharry III Emigrated to America in 1794*, (Lafayette, ID: Lafayette Printing Co., 1925)

183. Meharry Medical College, "1889 Meharry Medical College Catalogue," *Meharry Medical College Archives*, accessed December 22, 2015, http://diglib.mmc.edu/omeka/items/show/82.

184. "Walden University" (n. 180); "1889 Meharry Medical College Catalogue" (n. 183).

185. "Meharry Pharmaceutical College," *The Nashville Globe,* September 4, 1908, 17; Meharry Medical College, "1890 Meharry Medical College Catalogue," *Meharry Medical College Archives*, accessed March 3, 2016, http://diglib.mmc.edu/omeka/items/show/83. Meharry Medical College, "1899 Meharry Medical College Catalogue," *Meharry Medical College Archives*, accessed April 24, 2016, http://diglib.mmc.edu/omeka/items/show/92.

186. "1890 Meharry Medical College Catalogue" (n. 172).

187. Meharry Medical College, "1896 Catalogue," Meharry Medical College Archives, accessed December 27, 2015, http://diglib.mmc.edu/omeka/items/show/806.

188. "1890 Meharry Medical College Catalogue" (n. 172).
189. Meharry Medical College, "1899 Meharry Medical College Catalogue," *Meharry Medical College Archives*, accessed March 3, 2016, http://diglib.mmc.edu/omeka/items/show/92
190. "1889 Meharry Medical College Catalogue" (n. 68); Meharry Medical College, "1891 Meharry Medical College Catalogue," Meharry Medical College Archives, accessed March 3, 2016, http://diglib.mmc.edu/omeka/items/show/84
191. "1891 Meharry Medical College Catalogue" (n. 177)
192. "1896 Catalogue" (n. 174).
193. Charles Victor Roman, *Meharry Medical History: A History,* (Nashville, TN: Sunday School Publishing Board of the National Baptist Convention, Inc., 1934), 130
194. Meharry Medical College, "1922 Meharry Medical College Catalogue," *Meharry Medical College Archives*, accessed March 6, 2016, http://diglib.mmc.edu/omeka/items/show/111.
195. Meharry Medical College, "1929 Meharry Medical College Catalogue," *Meharry Medical College Archives*, accessed March 6, 2016, http://diglib.mmc.edu/omeka/items/show/118.
196. Roman, *Meharry Medical History: A History* (n. 193), 157, 160; *The Bulletin of the University of Minnesota, The College of Pharmacy Announcement for the Year 1919-1920, Vol. XXII No. 18 June 15, 1919*, (Minneapolis, MN: University of Minnesota, 1919); *The Bulletin of the University of Minnesota, The College of Pharmacy Announcement for the Year 1920-1921, Vol. XXIII No 24 June 19, 1920*, (Minneapolis, MN: University of Minnesota, 1920).
197. Roman, *Meharry Medical History: A History* (n. 193), 158.
198. Meharry Medical College, "1935 Meharry Medical College Catalogue," Meharry Medical College Archives, accessed December 23, 2015, http://diglib.mmc.edu/omeka/items/show/124.
199. Roman, *Meharry Medical History: A History* (n. 193), 160.
200. Roman, *Meharry Medical History: A History* (n. 193), 98.
201. Meharry Medical College, "1936 Meharry Medical College Catalogue," *Meharry Medical College Archives*, accessed March 3, 2016, http://diglib.mmc.edu/omeka/items/show/125.
202. Meharry Medical College, "1910 Meharry Medical College Catalogue," *Meharry Medical College Archives*, accessed April 3, 2018, http://diglib.mmc.edu/omeka/items/show/103
203. William L. Manggrum was another African American pharmacist who sponsored the *Cincinnati Manggrums*, a semi-professional baseball team, that

played in and around the Cincinnati, Ohio area in the 1940s on the Negro baseball teams circuit. It's not clear whether the team was a member of the National Association of Negro Base Ball Leagues (NANBL). William Manggrum was a 1921 graduate of the University of Pittsburgh College of Pharmacy and is reported to be the proprietor of the first black-owned drugstore in Cincinnati. See Lonnie Wheeler, "In the Shadows: Cincinnati's Black Baseball Players," in *The Cincinnati Game,* ed. Lonnie Wheeler (Wilmington, OH: Orange Frazer Press, 1988), 11-19; "Cincinnati Team to Play Pine Café Here Sunday," *The Newark Advocate*, August 14, 1948, 6. See also Gina Ruffin Moore, *Cincinnati* (Charleston, SC: Arcadia Publishing, 2007), 70.

204. Steve Pike, "The Martin Brothers," *WKNO 91.1,* April 29, 2014, https://www.wknofm.org/post/martin-brothers#stream/0; Earnestine Lovelle Jenkins, *Images of America: African Americans in Memphis,* (Mount Pleasant, SC: Arcadia Publishing, 2009), 40-41; Miriam DeCosta-Willis, *Notable Black Memphians*, (Amherst, NY: Cambria Press, 2008), 236-238.

205. Pike, "The Martin Brothers" (n. 204); "When Black Folks Owned Baseball Stadiums in Memphis: Dr. John B. Martin, The Martin Brothers & The Negro League," *Black History Heroes,* November 18, 2019, http://www.blackhistoryheroes.com/2018/06/when-black-folks-owned-baseball.html; "Martin/Martin's Stadium – Memphis TN," *Baseball Fever A Baseball Community,* November 20, 2019, https://www.baseball-fever.com/forum/general-baseball/ballparks-stadiums-green-diamonds/95848-martin-martin-s-stadium-memphis-tn

206. Pike, "The Martin Brothers" (n. 204); DeCosta-Willis, *Notable Black Memphians* (n. 204); Wikipedia contributors. "J. B. Martin." *Wikipedia, The Free Encyclopedia*. Wikipedia, The Free Encyclopedia, accessed March 1, 2016.

207. "Rival Parties Wage Battle for 3 Sanitary Board Posts," *Chicago Tribune,* October 24, 1952, 20; "Ex-sanitary Dist. Trustee Dies at 89," *Chicago Tribune,* May 2, 1973, 38.

208. "Negro Graduates in Medicine, Dentistry and Pharmacy – Commencement Exercises of Meharry Medical College," *The Tennessean*, February 9, 1894, 5; Meharry Medical College, "1894 Meharry Medical College Catalogue," *Meharry Medical College Archives*, accessed December 27, 2015, http://diglib.mmc.edu/omeka/items/show/87; Emma G. Wallace, "XI. Women in Pharmacy." *The Pharmaceutical Era,* 45 (1912): 702.

209. "Central Tennessee College," *The Nashville American,* September 24, 1898, 3.

210. Roman, *Meharry Medical History: A History* (n. 193), 14.

211. "The Negro in Pharmacy," (n. 2), p. 323.

212. Merlene Davis, "First Female Black Pharmacist No Longer Forgotten." *Lexington Herald-Leader,* February 8, 2009,

http://www.kentucky.com/2009/02/08/686969_first-female-black-pharmacist.html?rh=1; Merlene Davis, "Hidden History: Man's House Was Originally Home to City's First Black Female Pharmacist." *Lexington Herald-Leader,* February 8, 2009, B1.

213. Frank L. Mather, *Who's Who of the Colored Race: A General Biographical Dictionary of Men and Women of African Descent, Volume One 1915*, (Chicago, IL: Frank Lincoln Mather, 1915), 24; "Oklahoma board." *The Drug Circular,* 51 (1907): 575.

214. "National Council of Urban League Guilds: Frequently Asked Questions." *National Urban League.* Accessed March 3, 2016. http://nul.iamempowered.com/content/national-council-urban-league-guilds-frequently-asked-questions; Peter B. Flint, "Mollie Moon, 82, Founding Head of the Urban League Guild, Dies." *New York Times,* June 26, 1990, http://www.nytimes.com/1990/06/26/obituaries/mollie-moon-82-founding-head-of-the-urban-league-guild-dies.html; "National Urban League Guild President Mollie Moon Dies," *Jet,* July 16, 1990, 17.

215. "Artists of Johnson Brothers Third Annual Trade Show Named," *The Huntsville Mirror,* October 22, 1960, 4; "Clinic Spotlights Beauty Consultant, *Tampa Bay Times*, November 10, 1960, 23.

216. *Proceedings of American Conference of Pharmaceutical Faculties, Denver, Colorado, August 20-22*, 1912, (American Conference of Pharmaceutical Faculties, 1912), 85.

217. William C. Turner, "African-American Education in Eastern North Carolina: American Baptist Mission Work." *American Baptist Quarterly,* 12 (1992): 290-308.

218. W. H. Hartshorn, *An Era of Progress and Promise, 1863-1910,* (New York: The American Baptist Home Mission Society, 1890), 90.; Turner, "African-American Education in Eastern North Carolina" (n. 196).

219. *Sixth Annual Catalog of the Officers and Students of Leonard School of Pharmacy for the Academic Year Ending March 31, 1896*, (Raleigh, NC: Shaw University,1896); *Fifteenth Annual Catalog of the Officers and Students of Leonard Medical School, Shaw University, for the Academic Year 1894-95*, (Raleigh, NC: Shaw University, 1895).

220. *Sixth Annual Catalog of Officers and Students, 1896,* (n. 219).

221. It was not uncommon for pharmacy owners to deny African American pharmacy students the opportunity to acquire the necessary experiences for either graduation or registration as a pharmacist. See "The Negro in Pharmacy" (n. 2), 323; Lamb, *Howard University Medical Department, Washington* (n. 6), p. 46.

222. *Eighteenth Annual Catalog of the Officers and Teachers of the Leonard School of Pharmacy, the Pharmaceutical Department of Shaw University, Raleigh, North Carolina. For the Academic Year Ending May Thirty-First, Nineteen Hundred and Eight.* (Raleigh, NC: Edwards & Broughton Printing Co., 1908).

223. *Sixth Annual Catalog of Officers and Students, 1896,* (n. 219).

224. *Eighteenth Annual Catalogue of Officers and Teachers, 1908,* (n. 222).

225. Turner, "African-American Education in Eastern North Carolina" (n. 217), 301; Hartshorn, *An Era of Progress and Promise, 1863-1910* (n. 218), 88, 91.

226. *Fifteenth Annual Catalog of the Officers and Students* (n. 219).

227. "Death of William Simpson," *The Wilmington Messenger,* June 24, 1905, 3; William S. Powell, 1994 "Simpson, William," *NCpedia,* November 11, 2019, https://ncpedia.org/biography/simpson-william; "William Simpson, Wholesale and Retail Druggist," *Weekly State Journal*, April 6, 1880, 4.

228. "North Carolina Association," *The Druggist Circular,* (January 1907): 128-129.

229. "The American Pharmaceutical Association," *The Druggist Circular*, (January 1907); 100, 103.

230. "Board of Pharmacy," *The Druggist Circular*, (January 1907): 137, 144; "Pharmaceutical Association, The Twenty-First Annual Session Convened Here Yesterday," *The Semi-Weekly Messenger*, July 20, 1900, 8.

231. *Fifteenth Annual Catalog of the Officers and Students* (n. 219).

232. W. Conard Gass, 1979, "Battle, Herbert Bemerton," *NCpedia,* November 11, 2019, https://ncpedia.org/biography/battle-herbert-bemerton

233. *Annual Report of the North Carolina Agricultural Experiment Station, 18th Annual Report of the Director for 1895*, (Raleigh, NC: Ashe & Gatling, 1896).

234. "Battle, Herbert Bemerton" (n. 220); "Service for Dr. Battle," *The Selma Times-Journal,* July 4, 1929, 8.

235. *Eighth Annual Catalog of the Officers and Students* (n. 222).

236. *Annual Report of the North Carolina Agricultural Experiment Station, Annual Report of the Director for 1897 and 1898,* (Raleigh, NC: North Carolina Agricultural Experiment Station, 1898).

237. *Eighteenth Annual Catalog of the Officers and Teachers Sixth Annual Catalog of Officers* (n. 222).

238. *Eighteenth Annual Catalog of the Officers and Teachers Sixth Annual Catalog of Officers* (n. 222).

239. *Eighteenth Annual Catalog of the Officers and Teachers Sixth Annual Catalog of Officers* (n. 222); *Twenty-Second Annual Catalog of the Officers and*

Teachers of the Leonard School of Pharmacy, the Pharmaceutical Department of Shaw University, (Raleigh, NC: Shaw University, 1912).

240. *Sixth Annual Catalog of Officers and Students, 1896,* (n. 219).

241. Julia Pearl Hughes, an African American female pharmacist, tells of her experience in an article in the *Druggist Circular and Chemical Gazette,* 41 (November 1897):323, of being rejected for admission at Leonard School of Pharmacy on account of her gender.

242. "The Negro in Pharmacy" (n. 2), 323; *Eighth Annual Catalog of the Officers and Students of Leonard School of Pharmacy for the Academic Year Ending April 1, 1898*, (Raleigh, NC: Shaw University, 1898); "Commencement Exercises." *The Raleigh Daily Tribune* April 3, 1897, 5.

243. *Twenty-Second Annual Catalog of the Officers and Teachers of the Leonard School of Pharmacy,* (n. 239).

244. *Eighteenth Annual Catalog of the Officers and Teachers Sixth Annual Catalog of Officers* (n. 222).

245. Muskingum College (today Muskingum University) is a private liberal arts college, located in New Concord, Ohio. Founded in 1837, the predominant religious affiliation was with the Presbyterian Church, which reflected its Scotch-Irish heritage. In 1912, the College, after a unanimous vote of the faculty, awarded Dr. Shepard, the honorary Doctor of Divinity (D.D.) degree. At the time, he became the first African American in the history of the Muskingum College to receive a college degree. See also, Lenwood G. Davis, *Selected Writings and Speeches of James E. Shepard, 1896-1946, Founder of North Carolina Central University* (Madison, WI: Fairleigh Dickson University Press, 2013), 11; *Who's who in colored America* (Yonkers-on-Hudson, N.Y.: C.E. Burckel, 1933), 461; "Who Dr. Shepard Is," *The New York Age*, October 10, 1925, 3.

246. "Cuba Honors Dr. Shepard," *The Washington Bee*, February 5, 1910, 1; "Durhamnites in Cuba," *The Washington Bee*, February 5, 1910, 1; "National Religious Training School and Chatauqua/North Carolina Central University." North Carolina Central University, accessed February 12, 2020. https://www.opendurham.org/buildings/national-religious-training-school-and-chatauqua-north-carolina-central-university

247. "National Religious Training School" (n. 246); Charles W. Wadelington, "North Carolina Central University," North Carolina Central University *NCpedia*, accessed February 13, 2020, https://www.ncpedia.org/north-carolina-central-university;

248. "Our Heritage," North Carolina Central University, accessed February 9, 2020, https://www.nccu.edu/we-are-nc-central/our-heritage

249. *Who's who in colored America* (n. 245); "Native Born Hancock County Ga. African American Educators, Ministers, Medical," African American Bios, accessed February 12, 2020, https://georgriagenealogy.org/handcock2/aabios.html; Vivian Ovelton Sammons, *Black in Science and Medicine* (New York: Hemisphere Publishing Corp., 1990).

250. *Twenty-Second Annual Catalog of the Officers and Teachers of the Leonard School of Pharmacy,* (n. 239).

251. Ancestry.com. *U.S., Find A Grave Index, 1600s-Current* [database on-line]. Provo, UT, USA: Ancestry.com Operations, Inc., 2012.; Original data: *Find A Grave*. Find A Grave. http://www.findagrave.com/cgi-bin/fg.cgi.

252. Turner, "African-American Education in Eastern North Carolina" (n. 217), 290-308.

253. Turner, "African-American Education in Eastern North Carolina" (n. 217), 290-308.

254. Turner, "African-American Education in Eastern North Carolina" (n. 217), 290-308

255. Flexner, *Medical Education in the United States and Canada.* (n. 10).

256. Turner, "African-American Education in Eastern North Carolina" (n. 217), 290-308.

257. Todd L. Savitt, "Four African-American Proprietary Medical Colleges: 1888-1923," *Journal History Medical Allied Sciences,* 55.3 (2000): 203-255.

258. "1929 Meharry Medical College Catalogue," (n. 195).

259. "History." *History*. National Medical Association. http://www.nmanet.org/index.php/about-us/history, accessed March 26, 2016; "Dr. Miles V. Lynk." Tennessee History Classroom. http://www.tennesseehistory.com/class/Lynk.htm. Accessed March 26, 2016

260. "History" (n. 259); "Dr. Miles V. Lynk" (n. 259); "What the Negro is Doing: Matters of Interest Among the Colored People." *The Atlanta Constitution.* October 31, 1897, 32.

261. "Doctors Meet in 'Hub City': Eleventh Annual Convention of the N.M.A. in Session." *The Atlanta Constitution,* August 26, 1909, 1; "Colored Physicians Meeting in Columbus." *The Atlanta Constitution,* May 21, 1913, 3; "National Colored Medical Meet Here." *The Atlanta Constitution,* August 22,1920, 2.

262. Todd L. Savitt, 'A Journal of Our Own': The Medical and Surgical Observer at the Beginnings of an African-American Medical Profession in Late 19th-Century America, Part One." *Journal National Medical Association,* 88.1 (1996): 52-60.

263. "Colored Men and Women Wanted to Sell Lynk's Magazine." *Richmond Planet,* January 22, 1848, 2.

264. "Colored Men and Women Wanted" (n. 263).

265. Miles V. Lynk, *Sixty Years of Medicine: or The Life and Times of Dr. Miles v. Lynk, An Autobiography,* (Memphis, TN: Twentieth Century Press, 1951).

266. "Robert E. Hart: Founding Charter Member of the University of West Tennessee," in *Walking into a New Spirituality*, ed. Deacon Calvin S. Mcbride (New York: iUniverse, Inc., 2007), 23-31.

267. *Seventh Announcement of the Medical, Dental and Pharmaceutical Departments of the University of West Tennessee, Catalogue of 1906-7, Announcement for 1907-8,* (Memphis, TN: University of West Tennessee, 1907).

268. Savitt, "Four African-American Proprietary Medical Colleges: 1888-1923," (n. 257); Walking into a New Spirituality, (n. 266).

269. *Seventh Announcement of the Medical, Dental and Pharmaceutical Departments* (n. 267); *University of West Tennessee. College of Medicine and Surgery, Dental Surgery, Pharmacy, and Law, Catalogue for the Session of 1909-10, Announcement for the Session of 1910-11,* (Memphis, TN: University of West Tennessee, 1910).

270. *Seventh Announcement of the Medical, Dental and Pharmaceutical Departments* (n. 267).

271. *Seventh Announcement of the Medical, Dental and Pharmaceutical Departments* (n. 267).

272. *Seventh Announcement of the Medical, Dental and Pharmaceutical Departments* (n. 267).

273. *Seventh Announcement of the Medical, Dental and Pharmaceutical Departments* (n. 267).

274. Earnestine Lovelle Jenkins, *Images of America: African Americans in Memphis,* (Mount Pleasant, SC: Arcadia Publishing, 2009), 40-41; Miriam DeCosta-Willis, *Notable Black Memphians*, (Amherst, NY: Cambria Press, 2008), 236-238.

275. *Seventh Announcement of the Medical, Dental and Pharmaceutical Departments* (n. 267).

276. *Memphis Biography: George R. Jackson*. (Nashville, TN: Tennessee Historical Commission, 1990); *School of Pharmacy of the University of Michigan, Register of Alumni and Announcement, Twenty-six Year, 1893-1894*, (Ann Arbor: University of Michigan, 1893).

277. *Seventh Announcement of the Medical, Dental and Pharmaceutical Departments* (n. 261).

278. *Catalogue for the Session of 1909-10* (n. 269).

279. *Catalogue for the Session of 1909-10* (n. 269).

280. See Lovelle Jenkins. *Images of America* (n. 274).

281. It is uncertain when Beebe Steven Lynk was first appointed as Dean. The 1923 photo and the school's catalogues for 1907 and 1910 are the only documentation located at this time. Several volumes of the school's records have been missing for many years, which makes it difficult to establish when she started and how long she served as Dean. The significance of this appointment is that it raises questions that she may have been the first woman from a pharmacy degree program to serve as Dean over a pharmacy program in the U.S., and also whether the appointment as Dean included the other departments of the University.

282. *Seventh Announcement of the Medical, Dental and Pharmaceutical Departments* (n. 269), 9.

283. *The New York Age*, June 8, 1915, 6; *The New York Age*, June 22, 1916, 6.

284. "Fewer Newer Physicians," *The Bristol Herald Courier*, June 9, 1912, 4. See also, Savitt, "Four African-American Proprietary Medical Colleges" (n. 257); Flexner, *Medical Education in the United States* (n. 10).

285. Savitt, "Four African-American Proprietary Medical Colleges" (n. 257).

286. Savitt, "Four African-American Proprietary Medical Colleges" (n. 257); *Catalogue for the Session of 1909-10* (n. 269).

287. Savitt, "Four African-American Proprietary Medical Colleges" (n. 257); Lovelle Jenkins. *Images of America* (n. 274); DeCosta-Willis. *Notable Black Memphians* (n. 274).

288. *Seventh Announcement of the Medical, Dental and Pharmaceutical Departments* (n. 261).

289. *Catalogue for the Session of 1909-10* (n. 263).

290. Lovelle Jenkins. *Images of America* (n. 274).

291. New Orleans University. *Annual Catalogue of New Orleans University, 1904-1905, Thirty-Second Session,* (New Orleans, LA: Merchants Printing Co. LTD, 1905), http://hdl.handle.net/2027/uiuo.ark:/13960/t9h439v2b; Desha P. Rhodes, *A History of Flint Medical College, 1889 – 1911,* (Lincoln, NE: iUniverse, Inc., 2007), 15; New Orleans University. *Yearbook, Twenty-Eighth Session of New Orleans University, 1900-1901,* (New Orleans, LA: New Orleans University Print, 1901), http://hdl.handle.net/2027/uiuo.ark:/13960/t9h439v2b.

292. Rhodes, *A History of Flint Medical College* (n. 291).

293. Harry J. Meyers, *American College & Private School Directory, Vol. I,* (Chicago, IL: American Educational Association, 1907); Harry J. Meyers, *American College & Private School Directory, Vol. V.* (Chicago, IL: Educational Aid Society, 19ll), 136; Harry J. Meyers, *American College & Private School Directory, Vol. VI.* (Chicago, IL: Educational Aid Society, 1913), 139; Monroe N. Work, *Negro Yearbook and Annual Encyclopedia of the Negro, Tuskegee Institute, (*Tuskegee, AL: Negro Yearbook Co., 1913), 154.

294. Loyola University. *College of pharmacy (N.O.C.P.) Loyola University, Session Bulletin 1958. Vol. XL, No. 2.* (New Orleans, LA: Loyola University Bulletin, 1958).

295. "Loyola Closing Pharmacy School," *The Tuscaloosa News,* March 9, 1965, 4.

296. Carolyn Kolb, "New Orleans Pharmacists: A Story Worthy of a Museum." http://www.myneworleans.com/New-Orleans-Magazine/June-2014/New-Orleans-Pharmacists/. Accessed January 10, 2016.

297. *Yearbook, Twenty-Eighth Session of New Orleans University* (n. 291).

298. *Yearbook, Twenty-Eighth Session of New Orleans University* (n. 291).

299. J. H. Ford, *Caesar's Commentaries on the Gallic War and on the Civil War by Julius Caesar,* (El Paso, TX: El Paso Norte Press, 2005).

300. *Yearbook, Twenty-Eighth Session of New Orleans University* (n. 291).

301. *Yearbook, Twenty-Eighth Session of New Orleans University* (n. 291).

302. *New Orleans University Catalogue, 1911-1912,* (New Orleans, LA, 1912).

303. Miss Lucy Gonzales is listed in the first class of the Twenty-Eighth Session of the New Orleans University, 1900-1901 catalog, but is not listed in the graduating class of 1903. See *Yearbook, Twenty-Eighth Session of New Orleans University* (n. 291).

304. New Orleans University. Annual Catalogue of New Orleans University, 1904-1905, Thirty-Second Session. (New Orleans, LA: Merchants Printing Co. LTD, 1905). Accessed from: http://hdl.handle.net/2027/uiuo.ark:/13960/t9h439v2b.

305. *Annual Catalogue of New Orleans University, 1904-1905* (n. 304).

306. *Annual Catalogue of New Orleans University, 1904-1905* (n. 204).

307. "Minnie C. Moore." Year: 1920; Census Place: Chicago Ward 2, Cook (Chicago), Illinois; Roll: T625_307; Page: 1A; Enumeration District: 88; Ancestry.com. 1920 United States Federal Census [database on-line]. (Provo, UT, USA: Ancestry.com Operations, Inc., 2010).

308. Camille O. Green and Beebe Steven Lynk both graduated from a pharmacy program in 1903 and both were appointed as Professor of Pharmacy at their

respective alma mater that same year. With their appointments, it appears that they were the first African American women who graduated from a pharmacy degree program to serve on a pharmacy school faculty. See New Orleans University. *Annual Catalogue of New Orleans University, 1907-1908 Thirty-Fifth Session,* (New Orleans, LA: Merchants Printing Co., LTD, 1908); *Seventh Announcement of the Medical, Dental and Pharmaceutical Departments* (n. 267); *Catalogue for the Session of 1909-10* (n. 269). See also, *The Temple University Bulletin, Annual Catalogue 1911-1912* (Philadelphia, PA: Temple University, 1911), 325. It is not clear why she chose to acquire two of the same pharmacy degrees; "Mrs. Camille Mims." Ancestry.com. *U.S. City Directories, 1822-1995* [database on-line]. Provo, UT, USA: Ancestry.com Operations, Inc., 2011; "Thomas H. Mims." Year: *1920*; Census Place: *New Orleans Ward 3, Orleans, Louisiana*; Roll: *T625_619*; Page: *18B*; Enumeration District: *50*; See also, Emma Gray Wallace, "X. Women in Pharmacy," *The Pharmaceutical Era* (October 1912): 645-648.

309. Norman R. Smith, *Footprints of Black Louisiana* (Bloomington, IN: Xlibris Corporation, 2010), 39.

310. Pinckney Benton Stewart Pinchback was a politician during the Louisiana Reconstruction Era. He was the first African American to become governor of a state in the U.S.

311. "State Central Executive Committee Republican Party of Louisiana," *The Weekly Louisianan,* October 6, 1877, 2; "Emancipation Celebration," *The Weekly Louisianan*, September 10, 1881, 3; *Official Journal of the Proceeding of the House of Representatives of the State of Louisiana, The Regular Session, Begun and Held in New Orleans, January 7, 1878* (New Orleans, LA: The Office of the Democrat, 1878), 6-7.

312. Meharry Medical College, "1928 Meharry Medical College Catalogue," *Meharry Medical College Archives,* accessed November 22, 2019, http://diglib.mmc.edu/omeka/items/show/117

313. See Frank L. Mather, *Who's who of the Colored Race: A General Biographical Dictionary of Men and Women of African Descent, Volume 1* (University of California, 1915), 63

314. *Report of the Freedmen's Aid Society of the Methodist Episcopal Church* (Cincinnati, OH: R. F. Thompson, Printers, 1868).

315. Rhodes, *A History of Flint Medical College* (n. 285), 1-3.

316. Rhodes, *A History of Flint Medical College* (n. 285), 6-8.

317. "Negro Medical Colleges," *The New York Age*, July 7, 1910, 4; Flexner, *Medical Education in the United States and Canada* (n. 10); Harley, "The Forgotten History of Defunct Black Medical Schools" (n. 11).

318. New Orleans University. *Tan and Blue Catalogue Edition, New Orleans University, 1913-1914,* (New Orleans, LA: E. T. Harvey & Son, 1914), http://hdl.handle.net/2027/uiuo.ark:/13960/t7dr4fc96; New Orleans University. *Tan and Blue Catalogue Edition, New Orleans University, 1914-1915,* (New Orleans, LA: E. T. Harvey & Son, 1915), http://hdl.handle.net/2027/uiuo.ark:/13960/t85h9417m?urlappend=%3Bseq=3.

319. "Curing Aliments & Conquering Adversity: Flint-Goodridge Hospital 1896-1983," *Creolegen*, August 28, 2012, http://www.creolegen.org/2012/08/28/curing-ailments-conquering-adversity-flint-goodridge-hospital-1896-1983/

320. "Dillard Neighborhood Snapshot." http://www.datacenterresearch.org/pre-katrina/orleans/6/27/snapshot.html. Accessed 10 January 2016.

321. Henry McNeal Turner (1834-1915) was an author, civil rights activist, and a bishop of the African Methodist Episcopal (A.M.E.) Church. He was the first black man to hold the position of Chaplain in the U.S. Army. Turner served briefly in the Georgia State Legislature; and for twelve years he served as chancellor of Morris Brown College (now Morris Brown University) in Atlanta.

322. Booker T. Washington, 1856-1915, Educator; Washington was the foremost black educator of the late 19th and early 20th centuries. He also had a major influence on southern race relations and was the dominant figure in black public affairs from 1895 until his death in 1915. In 1881 he founded Tuskegee Normal and Industrial Institute (Tuskegee University today).

323. Dr. Thomas William Haigler was a physician, a surgeon, a pharmacist and an orator, he was also founder of the Chattanooga National Medical College.

324. *Catalogue of the Louisville National Medical College 1895-96, Eighth Annual Announcement,* (Louisville, KY: Ohio Falls Express Print, 1896).

325. *Sixteenth Annual Announcement, Louisville National Medical College, Departments of Medicine and Pharmacy, State University, 1903-1904,* (Louisville, KY: Louisville National Medical College, 1904).

326. *Sixteenth Annual Announcement* (n. 325).

327. *Nineteenth Annual Announcement of Louisville National Medical College, Department of Medicine and Pharmacy, State University, 1906-1907,* (Louisville, KY: The Franklin Printing Co., 1907).

328. *Nineteenth Annual Announcement* (n. 327).

329. *Sixteenth Annual Announcement* (n. 325); *Twentieth Annual Announcement of Louisville National Medical College, Department of Medicine and Pharmacy, State University, 1907-1908,* (Louisville, KY: The Franklin Printing Co., 1908).

330. *Sixteenth Annual Announcement* (n. 325).

331. *Sixteenth Annual Announcement* (n. 319); *Louisville National Medical College, Department of Medicine and Pharmacy, Fifteenth Annual Announcement 1902-1903,* (Louisville, KY: The Bradley & Gilbert Company, 1903).

332. *Sixteenth Annual Announcement* (n. 325).

333. *Sixteenth Annual Announcement* (n. 325).

334. *Fifteenth Annual Announcement* (n. 325).

335. *Catalogue Louisville National Medical College, 1897-98,* (Louisville, KY: Louisville National Medical College, 1898).

336. *Fifteenth Annual Announcement* (n. 331).

337. *Ninth Annual Report of the Indiana Board of Pharmacy. List of Registered Pharmacists and Registered Assistant Pharmacists Arranged Alphabetically and by Counties Alphabetically,* (Indianapolis, ID: Wm. B. Burford, Contractor for State Printing and Binding, 1908); See also, Ancestry.com. *U.S. Directories, 1822-1995* [database on-online]. Provo, UT, USA: Ancestry.com Operations, Inc., 2011.

338. "Firecracker" Case Decided. Mrs. Thelma Cole Loses Suit Against New Amsterdam Merchants." *The Courier-Journal* [Louisville] 24 Dec. 1914: 10. Print.

339. Otto L. Oppelt, *Gas Process*. United States Department of the Interior, Assignee. Patent 719,360, January 27, 1903; "Will Make Oil and Gas from Bituminous Shale. Patent of Dr. Oppelt." *The Courier-Journal,* January 29, 1903, 10; "Inventors rewarded with government patents." *The Courier-Journal, January* 28, 1903, 10.

340. "Patent of Dr. Oppelt" (n. 339); "Dr. Otto A. Oppelt Dies." *The Indianapolis News,* December 14, 1926, 7.

341. "Henry Fitzbutler: Medical School's First Black Graduate." *Michigan Alumnus,* 80.1 (1973): 29; M. M. Weiss, "History of Louisville National Medical College and the Red Cross Hospital: African American Medicine in Louisville, Kentucky – 1872-1976," *Louisville Medicine,* 60 (2012): 7-10.

342. *Fifteenth Annual Announcement* (n. 168); M. M. Weiss, "History of Louisville National Medical College and the Red Cross Hospital: African American Medicine in Louisville, Kentucky – 1872 to 1976, Part 2," *Louisville Medicine,* 61 (2013): 19-21.

343. "Documenting African American Life in Louisville: Newspapers. The Ohio Falls Express, July 11, 1891." http://louisville.libguides.com/c.php?g=158711&p=1040419. Accessed 12 May 2016.

344. George C. Wright, "William Henry Steward: Moderate Approach to Black Leadership," in *Black Leaders of the Nineteenth Century*, ed. Leon Litwack and August Meier. (Chicago, IL: University of Illinois Press, 1988), 275-285.

345. "Dr. Fitzbutler, the Colored Politician, Thinks That He is Elected to the School Board, as Mellet's Seat Was Vacant." *The Courier-Journal,* December 6, 1888; "Dr. Fitzbutler's Case." *The Courier-Journal,* December 18, 1883.

346. "The Meeting Called for Protest Against Dr. Fitzbutler's Becoming a Delegate is Not Held, but the Opposition Still Active." *The Courier-Journal,* April 17, 1884; "The Progress That is Being Made by the Colored Race in Louisville – Sketches and Anecdotes of Their Representative Men." *The Courier-Journal,* February 1, 1885, 1.

347. "The State Convention to Elect Delegates to the National Held Yesterday in Plymouth Church." *The Courier-Journal,* September 5, 1883; "A Lively Meeting Held at Armstrong Hall Last Evening to Appoint Delegates to the Richmond Convention." *The Courier-Journal,* April 27, 1884.

348. "Criminal Libel – Preacher Bates Causes the Arrest of Dr. Fitzbutler – Claims That False and Damaging Reports Were Published Concerning Him. *The Courier-Journal,* November 21, 1895.

349. "Couldn't Fire Him - Lively Meeting of the Republican City and County Executive Committee – the Attempt of the Willson Men to Expel Dr. Fitzbutler Fails." *The Courier-Journal,* December 1, 1888.

350. "State Board of Health Devoted Themselves to Dosing Irregular Brethren." *The Courier-Journal,* April 5, 1894, 6.

351. "Butchered – Awful Fate of Miss Flora Elliott – Betrayed by Her Lover – Brought Here from Indiana and Killed – by an Operation – Dr. Henry Fitzbutler, Colored, Arrested for Murder and Irvine M'coy as an Accessory." *The Courier-Journal,* June 5, 1898.

352. "Dr. Fitzbutler Dismissed." *The Courier-Journal,* June 17, 1898.

353. "Well-Known Colored Physician Dead – Dr. Henry Fitzbutler a Victim of Bronchitis Contracted While in England." *The Courier-Journal,* December 29, 1901, 2.

354. "Sued on State Taxes." *The Courier-Journal,* August 29, 1902, 1.

355. "Court Paragraphs." *The Courier-Journal,* March 20, 1904, 1; "Yesterday's Real Estate Transfers – Activity in Market Shown by Deeds Recorded in Courthouse." *The Courier-Journal,* July 29, 1908.

356. "Court paragraphs." *The Courier-Journal*, February 21, 1909, 1.

357. *Nineteenth Annual Announcement* (n. 321); Council on Medical Education and Hospitals (American Medical Association). *Medical Colleges of the United*

States and of Foreign Countries 1918, (American Medical Association, 1918), 10.

358. Savitt, "Four African-American Proprietary Medical Colleges" (n. 257).

359. It's uncertain whether Miss M.E. Jarman graduated. She is listed as the only pharmacy student in the *20th Annual Announcement of the Louisville National Medical College, 1907-1908*; however, records could not be found after 1908 that would help determine when she might have graduated.

360. Ancestry.com. *U.S. City Directories, 1822-1995* [database on-line]. Provo, UT, USA: Ancestry.com Operations, Inc., 2011.

361. "A Poor Snake Finds Whisky is Sure 'Cure'," *Chicago Tribune*, October 22, 1950, 246. "Secret Roster of Prohibition Agents Barred," *Chicago Tribune*, March 24, 1929, 26; "Jesse Merchant," *Chicago Tribune*, May 8, 1959, 62. See also, Frank L. Mather, *Who's Who in the Colored Race: A General Biographical Dictionary of Men and Women of African Descent, Volume One 1915,* (Chicago, 1915), 191.

362. William H. Ferris, "Frelinghuysen University of Washington Purchase and Moves Into New Building, *The Pittsburgh Courier,* February 19, 1927, 10.

363. *Courses of Study in the Frelinghuysen University of Washington, D.C.*(Washington, DC, Frelinghuysen University, 1920).

364. E. F. Harris, "Of Interest to Pharmacist: Another Pharmacy Course in D.C.," *Jour National Medical Assoc,* 11.4 (October-December 1919): 173.

365. Roy C. Darlington. *A History of Pharmaceutical Education at Howard University 1868-1981* (Xlibris: Howard University, 2016), 60.

366. "Boom Dr. Simmons for Education Board," *Washington Times,* April 20, 1919, 4; See also, "Colored Druggists to Meet," *Washington Herald*, January 14, 1919, 6.

367. Harris, "Of Interest to Pharmacists" (n. 364).

368. "Jesse Lawson is Dean; Served U.S. 44 Years, *Eastern Star*, November 6, 1927, 5.

369. "Decennial Catalogue of Frelinghuysen University" (2017). *Frelinghuysen Memorabilia*. 1. https://dh.howard.edu/ajc_freling/1 ; See "Anna Julia Cooper and Frelinghuysen University," *The House History Man,* February 18,2012, https://househistoryman.blogspot.com/2012/02/anna-julia-cooper-frelinghuysen.html.

370. *Courses of Study in the Frelinghuysen University* (n, 363).

371. "1922 Meharry Medical College Catalogue," (n. 194).

372. "New Drug Store for the Races," *The Tennessean,* January 27, 1918, 36; "Progress Among Colored People," *Aiken Standard*, December 3, 1924, 2;

Culp, *The Genesis of Black Pharmacists in America* (n. 52); "The Negro in Pharmacy" (n. 2), p. 323; Nicole Carmolingo, "Henry Rutherford Butler (1862-1931)" *New Georgia Encyclopedia,* accessed April 24, 2016, http://www.georgiaencyclopedia.org/articles/science-medicine/henry-rutherford-butler-1862-1931.

373. Thomas M. Morgan, "The Education and Medical Practice of Dr. James McCune Smith (1813-1865), First Black American to Hold a Medical Degree." *Journal National Medical Association.* 95 (2003): 603-613.

374. Culp, *The Genesis of Black Pharmacists* (n. 52); "The Negro in Pharmacy" (n. 2).

375. "Doctor L. L. Burwell." *Journal National Medical Association,* 20 (1928): 75; Wilhelmena S. Robinson, *International Library of Negro Life and History – the History of the Negro in Medicine,* (New York, NY: Publishers Company, Inc.,1967), 59-88.

376. Marilyn Pryce Hoytt, "Pryce's Pharmacy: Pouring Memories and Coke Generations." *Coca-Cola Journey,* N.p., 4 Feb. 2013. Accessed April 24, 2016, http://www.coca-colacompany.com/stories/pryces-pharmacy-pouring-memories-and-coke-for-generations/

377. Carmolingo, "Henry Rutherford Butler" (n. 372); Culp, *The Genesis of Black Pharmacists* (n. 52); "The Negro in Pharmacy" (n. 2).

378. "Color Line in Alabama." *The Pharmaceutical Era.* 13 (May 30, 1895): 674; Alabama Pharmaceutical Association. Proceedings of the Fourteenth Annual Meeting of the Alabama Pharmaceutical Association held at Montgomery. (Mobile, AL: Patterson & Hawes Printers, 1895).

379. American Pharmaceutical Association. *Proceedings of the American Pharmaceutical Association at the Forty-Third Annual Meeting held at Denver, Colorado, August, 1895.* (Baltimore, MD: American Pharmaceutical Association, 1895), 1148.

380. "Polk Miller," *The Pharmaceutical Era,* 11 (June 15, 1894): 577; "American Pharmaceutical Association," *The Pharmaceutical Era,* 11 (August 1, 1894): 125; "The Entertainments," *The Pharmaceutical Era,* 12 (September 15, 1894): 261; "Virginia Association," *The Druggist Circular and Chemical Gazette,* 41 (September 1897): 267.

381. "Richmond," *The Druggist Circular and Chemical Gazette,* 40 (January 1896): vii; "Polk Miller," (n. 88).

382. "A Bit of the South," *The Druggist Circular and Chemical Gazette,* 41 (March 1897): xxiii; "Trade Department," *The Pharmaceutical Era,* 12, no. 4 (August 15, 1894): 177; "Polk Miller," *The Druggist Circular and Chemical Gazette,* 36 (July 1894): 167.

383. "Polk Miller: An Unlikely African-American Music Historian," *NPR*: November 17, 2009, accessed June 24, 2018, https://www.npr.org/templates/story/story.php?storyId=120398673

384. "Doctors Meet." *The Washington Bee,* August 27, 1910, 1, 8; "Doctors Meet in Hampton, Virginia." *Nashville Globe,* September 1, 1911, 6; "Holds the Most Successful Meeting, at Hampton – Tuskegee Gets the Next Meeting." *The Washington Bee*, September 2, 1911, 1; J.P.H. Coleman, "Of Interest to Pharmacists," *Journal National Medical Association*, 4.1 (January-March 1912): 68; J. P. H. Coleman, "Proprietary Preparations vs Practical Pharmacy," *Journal National Medical Association*, 1.1 (January-March 1909): 4-9; J. P. H. Coleman, "To the Pharmacist," *Journal National Medical Association* 1.3 (July-September 1909): 170-171; "Doctors Meet." (n. 261); "Colored Physicians Ask that Additional Race Men be Made Commissioned Officers in the Army." *The New York Age,* September 7, 1918, 1; "Of Interest to Pharmacists. The Pharmaceutical Section," *Journal National Medical Association*, 8.2 (1918): 117; Delilah L. Beasley, "Pharmacists, Dentists and Doctors Meet," *Oakland Tribune,* July 21, 1931, 22.

385. Some of the socio-political and legal factors included: (1) Federal legislation prohibiting discrimination on the basis of race in employment and in education; (2) Federal legislation creating opportunities for minority groups in education; (3) Activism for change in discriminatory practices in education, employment, and in federal regulations; (4) Increases in federal funding that encouraged recruitment of more students in colleges of pharmacy; (5) Increases in the number of pharmacy schools nationally and for African-Americans; and (6) Professional associations and universities change in philosophy with more focus on diversity, gender, and inclusion.

386. "Our pharmaceutical colleges," *Drug Circular Chemical Gazette,* 41 (1897): 80-82.

387. *Proceedings of American Conference of Pharmaceutical Faculties, 1912* (n. 216).

388. *Catalogue of the University of Wisconsin 1896-97,* (Madison, WI: University of Wisconsin, 1897), p. 234. No practical experience was required for graduation if the student chose Graduate in Pharmacy (Ph.G.) degree program, which was a two- or three-year course. Students who chose the Bachelor of Science in Pharmacy (B.S.) degree program was required to complete practical experience to be awarded the degree.

389. *The University of Minnesota Bulletin, Vol. II, No.11, The College of Pharmacy* (Minneapolis, MN: University of Minnesota, 1899), p. 28; *The University of Minnesota College of Pharmacy 1909-1910, Volume XII, No. 3,* (Minneapolis, MN: University of Minnesota, 1909), p. 14; *The University of Minnesota College of Pharmacy 1914-1915, Volume XVII, No. 10,* (Minneapolis, MN: University of Minnesota, 1914), p. 7. The University of Minnesota awarded the

Pharmaceutical Chemist (Ph.C.) degree in 1899 around the same time the black pharmacy schools were awarding pharmacy degrees to the black students. Drug store experience was not required for graduation until the schools started awarding the B.S. degree in 1915.

390. *Register of Vanderbilt University for 1893-94 Announcement for 1894-95* (Nashville, TN: Vanderbilt University, 1894), p. 90-91. In the Department of Pharmacy at Vanderbilt, students in their Senior year, in the Pharmaceutical Chemist (Ph.C.) degree program, were required to complete a 10-week course in filing prescriptions. It appears that the University considered the experience comparable to drug store experience and enough for graduation. However, students enrolled in the Graduate in Pharmacy (Ph.G.) program were required to complete four years of practical experience in a drug store to be awarded the Ph.G. degree; see also "Our pharmaceutical colleges," (n. 371), p. lxxxii.

391. *Columbia University Bulletin of Information, College of Pharmacy of the City of New York included in Columbia University, July 1, 1904,* (Morningside Heights: NY: Columbia University, 1915), p. 10. The State of New York permitted graduates from recognized Schools of Pharmacy to take the licensing examination for the title of Junior Pharmacist if they were 19 years of age and have two years of experience in a drug store or registered pharmacy. The Board of Pharmacy counted the college courses toward meeting the experience requirement for examination.

392. "1891 Meharry Medical College Catalogue" (n. 190).

393. *Seventh Announcement* (n. 269); *Catalogue for the Session of 1909-10* (n. 269).

394. *Annual Catalogue of New Orleans University, 1907-1908* (n. 308); *Catalogue Louisville National Medical College, 1897-98* (n. 335).

395. *New Orleans University Catalogue, 1911-1912* (n. 302).

396. *Sixth Annual Catalog of Officers and Students, 1896,* (n. 219).

397. *Annual Catalogue of New Orleans University, 1907-1908* (n. 308).

398. "Conference of Faculties Meets: President Jordan Recommends Increasing Annual Dues, Carnegie Foundation Investigation of Schools, and Exchange Lectures," *Pharmaceutical Era* 52 (September 1919): 236-237.

399. Harley, "The Forgotten History of Defunct Black Medical Schools" (n. 11); Baker, "Creating a Segregated Medical Profession" (n. 11); Washington, "Segregation, Civil Rights, and Health Disparities" (n. 13); Robert B. Baker et. al., "African American Physicians and Organized Medicine, 1846-1968: Origins of a Racial Divide." *Journal of the American Medical Association* 300.3 (2008): 306-14. See also, Jasmine Arrington, "The Flexner Report and the African-American Health Experience Black Collective Memory and Identity as Shaped by Afro-cultural Trauma and Remembering," *Vanderbilt Undergraduate Research Journal,* 10 (Fall 2015): 1-8; Mark D.

Hiatt and Christopher G. Stockton, "The Impact of the Flexner Report on the Fate of Medical Schools in North America After 1909," *Journal American Physicians and Surgeons,* 8.2 (Summer 2003): 37-40.

400. Cooper, "The Negro in Pharmacy," (n 15). See also, Worthen, "Chauncey Ira Cooper" (n. 15).

401. Thompson, "Editorial Note" (n. 15).

402. "1920s Drugstore Gallery Cart," *North Carolina Museum of History,* January 12, 2020, https://www.ncmuseumofhistory.org/1920s-drugstore-gallery-cart

403. "African Americans in the Pharmaceutical Profession in the Mid-20th Century," (n. 56); "The Color Line in Pharmacy" (n. 52). For decades, white drug store owners would not service African-American patrons at their soda fountains and thus their drug stores became one of the major targets where protest took place throughout the 1960s' Civil Rights movement. See Booker, Jamal. "Fighting for Civil Rights at the Soda Fountain." http://www.coca-colacompany.com/history/fighting-for-civil-rights-at-the-soda-fountain (accessed January 14, 2018).

404. W. Michael Byrd and Linda A. Clayton. *An American Health Dilemma: A History of Blacks in the Health System, Beginnings to 1900* (New York, NY: Routledge, 2002), 373.

405. "1920s Drugstore Gallery Cart" (n. 387); "African Americans in the Pharmaceutical Profession in the Mid-20th Century," (n. 56). See also, W.A. "Bubba" McElveen, "A Look Back," *Sumter Item*, February 1, 2003; "Area Women Have Made Contribution," *Lifestyle*, March 26, 1988, 4.

406. Cooper, "The Negro in Pharmacy," (n. 34), p. 184.

407. Cooper, "The Negro in Pharmacy" (n. 34), p. 185. Other conclusions from the survey were: (4) That the average annual gross sales are adequate inducement to encourage ownership; (5) That the average value of stock and fixtures in these stores is approximately $12,000; (6) That employee (pharmacist) salaries are too low and there is need for better owner employee relationship; (7) That there are very few employees working in stores who anticipate studying pharmacy; (8) That the average owner is dissatisfied with the new graduate because, in his opinion, he lacks practical experience, has little desire to assume responsibility, and only wants to "fill prescriptions;" (9) That the average owner desires a graduate "well trained in practical pharmacy and the scientific principles of business;" (10) That there are a number of owners who feel that certain of their lay employees can be more important to their business than a pharmacist can be.

Index